Transforming Practice:

Life Stories of Transgender Men that Change How Health Providers Work

Marcus Greatheart MSW

Ethica Press

Toronto

Ethica Press
Toronto, Canada
ethica@ethicapress.com

Cover photo by Wayne Bund | waynebund.com

ISBN: 0991798902
ISBN-13: 978-0-9917989-0-2

DEDICATION

For my step-dad, Fred Dewar, who encouraged me to follow my academic dreams and to whom I am eternally grateful.

CONTENTS

Acknowledgements

I am deeply grateful to many people who helped me through the research and writing process: The FRED Study participants for their generosity in sharing their beautiful and fascinating stories; My graduate advisor, Dr. Brian O'Neill, for his guidance and belief in the importance of this work; Dr. Pilar Riaño-Alcalá for offering resources and support throughout this process; Dr. Aaron Devor for providing invaluable knowledge and insight; Drs. Amy Salmon and Beth Snow and the mentors and trainees at IMPART for their open minds and mutual passion for research; Michael Anhorn for his assistance with the focus groups, encouragement and comfortable sofa; Evie Erdmann and John Brennan for their love and friendship throughout this project; Chas Nol for helping keep my heart open; Marion Dewar, whose love and unwavering support makes her truly the best Mom ever; Tom Lampinen for believing in the researcher within me; Evin Taylor, Devon MacFarlane and the late Catherine White Holman for their unwavering support of this project; my friends, the many colleagues in trans work who have inspired me along the way. Special thanks to Geoff Watland for his amazing administrative support.

This research was funded in part by a fellowship from IMPART, the Integrated Mentorship Program for Addictions Research Training, and by a Masters Graduate Scholarship from the Canadian Institutes for Health Research.

1 | INTRODUCTION

There has been increased interest recently in issues relating to transgender communities, but much of the research and writing has been terribly dehumanizing and focuses almost exclusively on the problems these individuals experience, particularly in regard to mental health and substance abuse. My intent with this book is to provide an alternative view of transgender men, one that highlights their support systems, resources and competencies rather than the ongoing pathologizing that underscores present literature. In doing so I hope to present a more complex and nuanced exploration of gender transitions and transgender communities that brings those community members' voices back into the conversation.

Transgender People

Transgender people have existed throughout history and across numerous cultures, with many indigenous cultures recognizing some form of third gender individuals who are afforded great respect within tribal culture (Cole, Denny, Eyler & Samon, 2000). Susan Stryker (2008), among others, presents a fascinating and vibrant history of important transgender figures, researchers and clinicians, and describes the fight for transgender rights that continues to today (see also Lev, 2004). As both historical and contemporary transgender issues are made more challenging by the complexity of gender and its impact on individual and community experiences, discussion of these necessitates first reaching some agreement on language in order to talk and write about transgender people in a respectful way.

'Transgender' is considered by many an umbrella term that includes transsexuals, drag queens and kings, transvestites and genderqueers among a broad spectrum of individual identities and experiences that move among and between sex and gender categories (American Psychological Association, n.d.; Bockting, Robinson & Rosser, 1998). Sociologists Ekins and King (1999), in their grounded theory study of "cross-dressers and sex-changers" (p.580) incorporate three concepts of sex, gender and sexuality as they make operative a definition of 'transgendering' that "refers BOTH to the idea of moving across (transferring) from one pre-existing gender category to the other (either temporarily or permanently), AND to the idea of transcending or living 'beyond gender' altogether" (pp.581-582, original capitalization). Stephanie Brill (2009) uses 'transgender' more specifically to distinguish those who feel that their physical bodies do not represent their true gendered selves, whether or not they have chosen to adjust or change their gender presentation or undergo any medically-assisted gender reassignment. Brill, who works primarily with transgender and gender-variant children, consistently sets a clear boundary between discussions of gender and sexual identity, which may explain the desire to distance her work from the term 'transsexual' for having the word 'sex' within it.

The American Psychological Association (n.d.) describes 'transsexuals' as "transgender people who live or wish to live full time as members of the gender opposite to their birth sex" (p.3). Inherent in this definition are problematic assumptions of a gender binary and a complete transition. This Association states that transsexuals usually seek hormones and surgery to make their bodies as congruent as possible with their preferred sex; this language highlights and thus privileges a prescribed route of medical interventions over the individual and social experience of transition. The dominant medical literature tends to use 'FTM' (female-to-male) or 'female transsexual' in its categorization of these individuals (Forshee, 2008); the former provides information that may be useful in certain medical situations, while the latter is confusing to anyone but the psychiatric professionals who use it. When quoting others I use their terminology.

In this book I use the term 'transgender' differently. I recognize multiple genders, rather than just two, and suggest that these might be most easily understood as points across a continuum of gender. I use the term 'transgender (or trans) man' to refer to individuals whose sex was identified as female at birth, were socialized as girls and women, and are now living as guys or men on the transmasculine gender continuum; in this way I honour the 'affirmed' or expressed gender of these men. Similarly, I use the term 'transgender (or trans) woman' to refer to individuals who were identified as male at birth, socialized as boys and men, and are now living on the trans-feminine spectrum of gender expression.

The population size of transsexuals and transgender people has also been the subject of much debate, in part due to the differences in language and definition. In light of the broad definitions of transgender, some have attempted to assess the prevalence of trangenderism, as defined by the American Psychiatric Association (2000), as not a particularly common phenomenon and thereby dismissing these groups as small and insignificant (Lev, 2004). The American Psychiatric Association, in its current *Diagnostic and Statistical Manual of Mental Disorders* [DSM-IV-TR] (2000), lays out four criteria for individuals diagnosed with Gender Identity Disorder (GID) as:

    a) "strong and persistent cross-gender identification",

    b) "persistent discomfort with [natal] sex or sense of inappropriateness in the gender role of that sex",

c) "disturbance...not concurrent with physical intersex condition", and

d) "disturbance causing significant distress or impairment in social, occupational, or other important areas of functioning" (code 302.85). These criteria limit the range of people under the umbrella of 'transgender' to those meeting a particular diagnosis defined by a dominant medical institution.

The updated *DSM-V*, expected later this year, will replace GID with Gender Dysphoria (GD), with adjusted definitions and criteria.

Regardless of the criteria, the number of transsexuals has yet to be identified with any certainty. The *DSM-IV-TR* (2000) states that one in 100,000 females (FTM) and one in 30,000 males (male-to-female transsexuals) undergo gender reassignment. Seil (2004) reports that the prevalence is higher in countries where treatment is more readily accessible and acceptable. In the Netherlands, where transsexuals may have easier access to surgeons and other care providers, transsexualism is seen in one in 11,900 MTF and one in 30,400 FTM people (Meyer et al., 2002), again based on those seeking gender reassignment. As dickey (2009) points out, this suggests a ratio of one FTM for every three MTF individuals.

Conway (2002) reported significant errors in the prevalence numbers used in the *DSM-IV-TR*. She and others (Human Rights Campaign, 2006) report that the prevalence numbers used in the *DSM-IV-TR* date back to the 1960s when far fewer people were coming forward as transsexual and, further, represent only those who have sought out surgical interventions. For many years she has documented the number of specifically MTF gender reassignment surgeries (GRS) conducted by physicians in the United States and used these figures to estimate the prevalence of MTF GRS to be about one in 2,500. Further, she states that the prevalence of transgender individuals (non-operative) is one in about 500 adult males (Conway, 2002). Using Conway's calculations and the ratio of one FTM for every three MTF individuals, dickey (2009) suggests that one in every 8,350 adult females (FTM) have completed GRS and about one in 1,675 adult females (FTM) is transgender. There is no simple way to accurately determine the prevalence rates of this burgeoning community, (dickey, 2009; Lev, 2004).

Further, dickey (2009) explored the possibility of counting the number of FTM people as those who opt for 'top surgery,' a form of mastectomy with chest contouring. He states that top surgery is the only procedure most FTM people choose to have and yet, the number of plastic surgeons, gender clinics and general surgeons who offer the procedure make it difficult to calculate the number of people who get it done.

Further complicating the calculation is that most insurance providers in the United States will not cover the cost of any GRS procedures. As a result, anecdotal reports state that some surgeons in the United States and Canada have offered to perform radical mastectomies on trans men with no insurance coverage. Unfortunately this removes the entire breast tissue and often leaves unsightly scarring and malformation of the chest. More desirable is chest contouring surgery which retains some breast tissue to create a more masculine chest appearance. Furthermore, other reports suggest that hysterectomies are sometimes done under the guise of another pathology and thus requiring a more aggressive surgery than necessary. Wilson (2005) lists a total of six U.S. employers that allow for inclusion of GRS procedures as a part of their standard health care coverage. I found no estimates of the numbers of trans surgeries performed in Canada, but will discuss later the state of trans healthcare here.

Recent Issues in Transgender Health

In the last few years, activists and clinicians in North America have been debating the forthcoming fifth edition of the *DSM* (Drescher, 2009) expected in May 2013. It will replace the *DSM-IV-TR* (American Psychiatric Association, 2000) is presently the dominant resource used by mental-healthcare providers in North America to describe and treat mental illness. According to Peter Rothberg (2008), journalist and blogger for *The Nation*, of particular concern to trans-allied individuals was the especially contentious appointment of Kenneth Zucker of the Centre for Additions and Mental Health in Toronto to co-chair the committee overseeing this review; Zucker is often accused of being a proponent of 'reparative therapy' for transsexualism among children and youth who demonstrate gender-variant behaviours and/or assert their gender to be discordant with the sex they were determined to be at birth. Although there is a lack of evidence to support these accusations, activists worried that Zucker's leadership of the committee would result in the *DSM-V* recommending reparative therapy (Rothberg, 2008) and, further, categorizing transsexualism as a form of homosexuality (Drescher, 2009). That does not seem to be the case.

Trans woman and author Julia Serano (2009) cautioned about presenting an 'us vs. them' conflict over the *DSM-V* committee appointments and the resulting debate during her keynote address to the Philadelphia Trans-Health Conference:

> In certain sexology circles, the negative reactions expressed by trans activists in response to these incidents have been caricatured as expressions of narcissistic rage[1]—a hysterical, irrational, mass overreaction to the supposedly logical, well-reasoned, empirically-based theories and diagnoses forwarded by psychologists. Reciprocally, in trans circles, psychologists are sometimes caricatured as heartless evil-doers who conspire behind the scenes in order to figure out how to further exploit and subjugate trans people via the *DSM*, WPATH [World Professional Association for Transgender Health] *Standards of Care*, and so on, in order to achieve academic success and/or monetary gain for themselves. (n.p.)

---

[1] I thank Aaron Devor for identifying the term "expressions of narcissistic rage" as one attributed to Anne Lawrence, a noted MTF trans researcher and advocate.

These camps are far from definitive as there are many psychologists and other mental-health providers with great competence who work with trans people. Serano sees the difference as those willing to hear and accept that trans people have much to say and inform discussions of gender and their own care in contrast to those who dismiss the voices of trans people. Still others, like Serano, wanted to see transsexualism removed completely from the *DSM-V*, and instead address the health needs of trans people as more generalized physical health issues. The APA appears to have made a gesture in this direction with their decision to replace GID with GD.

Broadly, the present literature about trans men includes legal papers, historical papers, sociological and anthropological works, and a growing body of medical and psychological literature written by trans professionals. There is also a medical literature focused on GID, the mental illness described previously that provides rationale for treatment, some of which will need to be revised in light of the emergent GD recategorization. Missing from most of the literature are the description and analysis of the spectrum of practical resources that trans communities and service providers can access. As the late trans activist Kyle Scanlon (2006) reminds us:

> For too many trans folks ... being trans hasn't been an opportunity for subverting the patriarchy or playing with gender. Instead, being trans has meant fighting for survival, recognition, equality, housing, employment, safety and medical care. (p.88)

There is a need to understand better both the strengths and barriers trans people face in meeting basic needs and to use this knowledge to inform 'best practices' for service providers working with them. This book intends to fill this gap. As I will discuss in the next chapter, there are real concerns for the health of trans men. While the origins of these issues are disputed – whether forged in mental illness or a result of social stigma – the reality is that service providers need to address these concerns in practice today, while working to ensure equitable and appropriate access to healthcare in the future.

As health professionals, we often work in mental-health and addictions-support capacities and may need to assist clients to unpack the role that gender may or may not play in the challenges they face. As generalist practitioners working in hospitals or community-based agencies, we will likely encounter individuals who are trans or who are gender variant in presentation. An investment in social justice requires us to be not just aware of transgender issues, but to conduct an assessment of how our programs are gendered and how a transgender person would be supported or blocked in accessing services. We must be prepared to interpret the social needs of trans clients to other health professionals. At the end of an hour-long in-service for healthcare providers I conducted a few years ago, a physician bluntly dismissed the necessity of the training stating the clinic absolutely did not have any transgender patients. Considering the efficacy of hormones and GRS for some individuals, I asked how clinic personnel would even know if a client was transgender. Some professionals and non-professionals alike seem to think they have the ability to visually identify every trans person, which is simply not the case. Levels of bias and misinformation are high among health care professionals and specialized training to work with a transgender population is far less frequent (Carroll & Gilroy, 2002). In fact, Sanchez (2002, cited in Maguen, 2005) states that the insensitivity of health care providers is the primary reason why transgender people do not access services. In my experience, new and current trans clients only begin emerging once a clinic or program creates a welcoming, trans-competent environment.

My Personal Connection to Trans Health and Wellness

On a road trip along the West Coast of the United States from May to July 2007, I met a number of trans men, many of whom are now good friends. As a person with a longtime interest in gender and its impacts on peoples' lives and social interactions, I listened intently as these men shared their stories. One friend spoke of his teenaged years when, on a monthly basis and coinciding with his menstrual cycle,[2] he would "get crazy, get wasted and fuck around." On reflection he said he could ignore what was in his underwear rather effectively most of the time, but he was unable to cope with the physical manifestations of menstruation. Another friend spoke about

---

[2] Here I use a masculine possessive pronoun in reference to menstruation to honour the affirmed gender of the individual who shared the story, thus creating a conflict of gendered language that often happens when writing about and working with trans people.

the challenges of dating as a queer trans man in a phallocentric gay community. His politics of disclosure were considered radical by many of our friends — he would not reveal being trans until absolutely necessary or not at all — and as a result more than a few of us were concerned for his safety. Yet another recalled the absurd, unsympathetic and often degrading interactions he had endured with healthcare providers as he negotiated the obstacle course of medically-supported gender transition; sadly these stories are far too commonplace among the many trans people with whom I have spoken since. There were many other stories about the challenges trans men have faced and yet, despite these, they seemed generally well-adjusted and content with their lives.

These stories still echoing through my head, I surveyed the extant literature for research that explored mental health and wellness among trans men. I was operating with the Canadian Mental Health Association's (n.d.) definition of 'mental health' as a measure of life enjoyment, resilience in the face of stress or challenges, balance among different areas of life, self-actualization of our abilities and strengths to reach our full potential, and the flexibility to balance emotions and expectations. While the literature was small, I did find a number of psychiatric articles that presented trans men only as sufferers of mental illness (Cole, O'Boyle, Emory and Meyer, 1997; Lobato, Koff, Manenti, Salvador, da Graça, Petry, et al., 2006), an image that was a stark contrast to that of my friends. Many of the reports linked this so-called 'illness' to depression, substance abuse and suicide; here, there was even less resonance to the people I had met. As I looked deeper, I discovered an even smaller collection of articles, books and clinical guidelines, written by trans people and non-transgender allies, that began to resemble the narratives I had heard on my journey (Devor, 1997; Lev, 2004).

Having identified a clear gap in the literature and resources, and concurrently receiving support from friends and professionals working within trans communities, I decided to focus my graduate research on learning more from, and then sharing, the stories of trans men who are contented with their lives despite, and often in appreciation of, the challenges they have experienced in their lives. My intent remains that, by activating a critical lens within this research, I can provide for my professional colleagues and our allies some recommendations for effective and culturally appropriate practice with trans communities. More importantly, I hope that my findings will improve the future experiences of trans men who decide to employ our support and care as they consider, initiate and progress through an important stage in their lives: transition.

My own social locations

As a non-trans queer man I was at first skeptical of my capacity as a community outsider to successfully conduct such a project. Would my work scream of biocentrism? Would my class, education and white-male privilege negatively impact the work? Perhaps another trans man should do this. Yet many discussions with community members and service providers revealed the need for informed, non-trans allies to support the movement toward social justice for trans people. As an anti-oppressive researcher, I take seriously the advice of University of Victoria social work researchers Karen Potts and Leslie Brown (2005) to engage in ongoing reflection, critique and challenge my research process and the resulting knowledge production in order to transform research, practice, and society (p.260). Moreover, my goal with this project is to "construct emancipatory, liberatory knowledge that can be acted on, by, and in the interest of the marginalized and oppressed" (p.262) who are, in the case of this project, trans communities.

In order to be transparent about how I bring particular experiences and perspectives to this work, I recognize myself as narrator and primary author of this work. I am a queer man, trans ally and social worker; these social locations both inform and bias my analysis and re-presentation of the stories of trans men within this report. Further, I recognize how these locations can create a chasm between research participants and myself as researcher; Fine (1994) refers to this dynamic as the Self-Other dichotomy. Commenting on Fine's work, Ester Madriz (1998) explains: "Whereas the Self often represents what is middle class, White, and often male, the Other is often identified with the colonized – women and men of color, poor people, gays and lesbians, and individuals with disabilities" (p.115). In order to counter this dichotomy Madriz recommends researchers create environments in which they stand with, rather than in opposition to, oppressed groups. In my approach to this work with trans men, and in each interaction, I made every effort to reduce the impacts of these relational differences.

I bring attention to some of the mistakes I have made along the way not only in the interest of transparency, but also to share the learning I take from these errors that future researchers may find helpful to avoid similar pitfalls. I have made efforts to vet the stories in this book through many conversations with trans men at conferences and in my own social network. I also shared these with the members of the project Advisory Group, local trans men who provided valuable insights during development, deployment and analysis of this project. I alone take full responsibility for any inaccuracies and errors contained herein.

As a community-involved individual, my anecdotal experience has been that most people find trans issues unfamiliar, curious, and sometimes highly uncomfortable. There is little information available in general society about trans communities and what does exist, is often inaccurate. My own investment in trans issues developed as I met more and more trans men within my own social circles and in my counselling practice. I took it upon myself to learn more about trans people's experiences so that I could be a better friend, care provider, and ally. Ally-ship honours the integrity of trans individuals and their communities and keeps in mind the words of Kyle Scanlon (2006) that a "trans ally is someone willing to stand up and fight for the basic human rights and dignity of all trans people" (p.88).

We must keep in mind the history our trans clients may have had at the hands of other less-competent providers (Raj, 2002) and the resulting distrust. We all hold some of the responsibility for that distrust; as a non-trans person, a citizen, and a healthcare provider, I recognize that I have contributed to the ongoing oppression of trans and gender-variant people. Most all of us have used language that perpetuates the discrete categorization of behaviour, appearance and gender performance, and in so doing marginalized and in some instances perpetuated the gender binary. These are the burdens that all providers share, regardless of their gender identity.

With this project I present pragmatic recommendations for health practice that can both facilitate transition for trans people, and encourage competent generalist practice with all gender-variant clients. To that end, my framework for inquiry draws on a strengths-based model (Saleebey, 1996; Graybeal, 2004) more typically used in social work practice to inform my social work research. From this perspective I take issue with a medical literature that identifies deficiencies within trans communities, while rarely highlighting strengths.

Assumptions

Despite implications of pathology subsumed within a psychiatric diagnosis, I assume that it is possible for a trans person to lead a happy life and, where a trans man reports having a happy life, I accept that self-report at face value. I assume the necessity of a critique of the medical institution as a whole and how medicine is practiced and performed. Within this critique an evaluation of the way transsexuals and trans people fall under the mental illness rubric as defined by the American Psychiatric Association's diagnostic criteria is necessary. I come to this work with a belief that trans men have something of value to share with our communities and I bring an openness to support people who are exploring, shifting, or changing their gender. My belief as a health provider and researcher is that trans men are not mentally ill solely on the basis of being trans, despite the appearance of such as a result of GID or GD appearing within the *DSM*. I do not deny that trans people are at risk for the same mental illnesses as a non-trans person, and may be more susceptible to mental illnesses related to the stress they experience due to discrimination and marginalization. Finally, by hearing stories of satisfaction I recognize the possibility of affecting change and perhaps enhancing the lives of trans men.

Context

The appearance of openly trans people in the social context has been a relatively recent event. A number of authors have offered in-depth studies of trans people in society that I will not attempt to recreate here (see Cole, Denny, Eyler and Samon, 2000; Devor, 1997; Lev, 2004; Stryker, 2008). Trans people have often been socially situated within lesbian and gay communities and assumed to be a homogeneous group despite unique differences between gender and sexual identities; sexuality and gender are often conflated thus creating confusion for many in everyday conversation (Forshee, 2008). The experiences of trans people as discussed in the professional literature is often located within health institutions and limited to those where surgical procedures take place. This is a site of medical intervention for trans people and, therefore, part of the social experience of transition. The lack of standardization in the provision of services can add to the tenuousness of the experience. Fortunately, this is also the place where we can operate as allies. Unfortunately, the relationship between trans people and their healthcare professionals remains a contentious one as a result of providers who have operated with questionable ethics and used their 'gatekeeper' status to enforce gender-normative behaviours and participation in demeaning research protocols (Raj, 2002).

Even within the problematic medical milieu where diagnostic options and treatments are delineated, many transgender people struggle to access the care that is prescribed therein. A survey of the trans healthcare landscape is helpful here. In Vancouver, Canada, a gender clinic at Vancouver General Hospital provided assessment and treatment of individuals diagnosed with GID until 2002. According to Vancouver Coastal Health (VCH) (2009), this clinic was part of the Centre for Sexual Medicine and offered its patients "endocrinological, urological/gynecological, psychiatric, psychological, and social services, and was the sole gatekeeper for public health coverage for transition-related surgeries." The program ended when provincial budget cuts forced the Department of Psychiatry at the hospital to reduce the program size. As a result, clinic staff felt they could no longer provide service to transgender people. After the closure of the clinic, a community consultation lead to the development of what is now the Transgender Health Program (THP) also offered through VCH. The THP provides referrals, resources and training on a range of topics for both trans-community members and service providers.

Elsewhere in British Columbia there are specialists who offer some trans-specific services, and the THP often provides training to ensure the competence and cultural capacities of these professionals. Across Canada, the Sherbourne Health Centre in Toronto has a reputation within trans communities for offering trans-sensitive service, while the Centre for Addictions and Mental Health (CAMH) in the same city has a more conflicted history with trans communities. In Montreal, the GRS Clinic has a long history of providing surgical care for transgender people.

Many of my American friends and colleagues are of the opinion that Canada's universal healthcare means trans people have significantly easier access to transition-related interventions that are paid by the state. While the situation does indeed seem somewhat better in that some degree of coverage is available in some jurisdictions, access is still highly problematic in many ways for a majority of trans people.

Coverage of gender reassignment treatment by medical insurance plans varies among provinces and territories. Variations include: which surgeries are covered; the amount of coverage, which often does not cover the full cost of procedures; and whether surgical assessments and the procedure are provided in- or out-of-province. British Columbia has its own surgical assessors, and provides some coverage of some GRS surgeries.

For trans men, chest contouring surgery is now covered in British Columbia but phalloplasty is not. For trans women, the costs for penectomy, orchiectomy and vaginoplasty are covered at GRS Montreal; individuals must cover their own accommodations and travel costs. The province has a trained surgeon who could provide all necessary GRS-related surgeries, however the provincial government will not provide use of public surgical facilities (CPATH, 2011).

According to Knudsen and Corneil (2009), the terrain varies across the country: Alberta formerly covered all surgeries for up to 16 individuals a year, but cut all funding to GRS in April 2009 resulting in a Human Rights Commission complaint (CBC, 2009). In Saskatchewan and Manitoba, trans people must travel to CAMH in Toronto for surgical assessment; some surgeries are provided in province while the rest are performed at GRS in Montreal where only direct surgical costs (about 25% of total cost) are covered. As a result of a Human Rights Commission ruling, Ontario began providing full coverage for transgender surgeries as of June 2008. CAMH currently provides assessments although other community groups are attempting to expand access to assessments. In Quebec, hysterectomy is provided by many in-province surgeons while other surgeries such as chest surgery, metoidioplasty and and phalloplasty are usually referred to GRS Montreal. New Brunswick, Nova Scotia and Prince Edward Island have trained assessors as of 2008 but the provinces will not provide coverage of surgeries; a group is lobbying to change this. While in Newfoundland and Labrador surgeries are apparently covered after assessment at CAMH, no one has yet received any of the surgeries. Information regarding GRS coverage in Nunavut, the Yukon and Northwest Territories was unavailable.

There are further structural challenges related to transition in terms of jurisdictions that require surgery in order to change the gender on a birth certificate. For example, in British Columbia, section 27 of the *Vital Statistics Act* (1996) requires evidence of "trans-sexual surgery" in the form of a letter from the surgeon who performed it, and a physician within the province who has examined the individual affirms that "the trans-sexual surgery is complete by accepted medical standards." A trans man might not want to have surgery and also not want to live with a driver's license that categorizes him as female. As a result he might feel pressured towards surgery and forced to decide what is more important: having the gender category on his driver's license represent him accurately or accept the risks of unwanted surgery.

Delimitations

This book focuses on a particular group of trans men and may not be generalizable in a statistical sense to other trans men. That stated, these findings might still be useful and contribute to understanding issues in serving other trans men. I do not explore the experiences of trans women; while some of the issues may be similar, neither the methodology nor the analysis of the data considered the trans-feminine spectrum. Generalization from the findings of this study to the trans-feminine spectrum would, therefore, be problematic.

This is a book about gender and not about sexuality, two concepts that have historically been conflated (Forshee, 2008), perhaps due to the so-called lesbian, gay, bisexual and transgender (LGBT) community and the inferred affinity between these groups. Stryker (2008) recounts in her book *Transgender History* numerous intersections, often under the banner of united protest and celebration. There was the riot in San Francisco at Compton's Café in August of 1966 when the "usual late-night crowd of drag queens, hustlers, slummers, cruisers, runaway teens, and down-and-out [Tenderloin] neighborhood regulars" responded to ongoing aggressive police behaviour with a barrage of dish and tableware and fighting on the street (pp.64-65). Almost three years later in New York City, trans people and their gay and lesbian compatriots fought a similar battle against harassment in front of the Stonewall Inn. More recently there are LGBT pride parades in most Western cities nowadays, and trans and queer people are working together within organizations such as EGALE, Lambda Legal and the Gay and Lesbian Task Force to further rights for all sexual- and gender-minority people. Relations between these groups have endured a long history of tumult and celebration, and yet we cannot allow this relationship to confuse the unique differences between them. This book is focused very specifically on experiences of gender and not on the stories that the men share about their sexual identity. This is not to deny kinship between trans people and lesbian and gay people that has emerged from a long mutual history of shared oppression, but my approach honours many people's lived experience that gender identity and sexual orientation are separate issues.

This book intends to bring a critical lens to the stories trans men share about their transition experiences and post-transition lives, and what makes them content. In doing so, I intend to highlight individual and social experiences of transition over the medicalized ones. In the interest of being transparent about the critical lens I bring this work, in the next chapter I explore the theoretical literature first and the medical afterward. In Chapter 3, I share the stories of eight generally-satisfied trans men and, finally in Chapter 4 provide a discussion of the findings in relation to current research and theory, their implications for healthcare practice, and future directions for research.

2 | CONCEPTUAL CONTEXT

This chapter is divided into three parts. In *Theoretical Underpinnings*, I begin with an exploration of the history of 'transgender' in feminist theory and a discussion of trans-feminist theory, the lens through which I undertook this project. Then I present models for the assessment of life satisfaction and well-being, and relate these to recent literature on quality-of-life of trans people. In *Theoretical Identity Frameworks*, I look at identity from two perspectives: the first involves two complementary models of trans-identity development, while the second explores and critiques how transgender identity is created in the extant health and mental health literature. In *Implications for Practice*, I discuss the role of the health professional in transgender care, and conclude with an explanation of strengths-based practice studying relation to this work.

THEORETICAL UNDERPINNINGS

The utility of feminism in transmasculine studies

Much like contemporary Canadian artists attempting to represent our geographic landscape will always need to respond to the canonical Group of Seven artists, the feminist perspectives on the 'transgender issue' will forever be obliged to engage with the vehement protests of radical feminist Janice Raymond. In 'The Politics of Transgender' (1994), an update to her influential book *The Transsexual Empire* (1979), Raymond heartily singles out trans women who are not "real women" but rather "patriarchal...stereotypes of femininity" (p.628). According to Raymond, trans women are drag queens and appropriators of women's gender performance; as an essentialist, Raymond refuses to acknowledge anyone who is not a natal woman. In light of her categorical organization of gender, it surprises me that Raymond basically ignores trans men in her analysis by essentially grouping them with natal women based on her criteria.

Interestingly Raymond privileges those trans people who engage with the medical establishment and undergo sex reassignment surgery; these are the "true transgenderists" (p.629), compared to those who just use hormones. She not only reveals her ignorance about the need for ongoing, post-surgical, endocrine therapy, but also exposes a decidedly curious support of the patriarchal medical institution that is complicit in the pathologizing of trans and other gender-variant people. Finally, when Raymond decrees that "transgenderism reduces gender resistance to wardrobes, hormones, surgery and posturing – anything but real sexual equality" (p.632), she denies trans people their subjective experience of internal/external dissonance and their goal of finding a place of honour for themselves in a society where hegemonic ideals about sex and gender dominate each and every one of us.

What are Raymond and her radical feminist compatriots so afraid of? Surya Monro and Lorna Warren (2004) contend that the artillery is out because the battle is foundational:

> Transgender poses a serious theoretical challenge to feminism. Feminisms, particularly radical feminism, are based on the notion of an unequal gender-binaried system. Transgender scrambles gender binaries and opens up the space beyond or between simple male-female categorization. It also highlights the flaws in...the simplistic equation of masculinity with oppression. (pp.354-355)

Having reviewed this literature, I challenge radical and other essentialist feminists' anti-trans criticisms: What are the categories that make a woman? Some suggest biology and sociology, nature or nurture, or hormones and female reproductive organs. But are women limited to XX chromosomes? Must women be raised and socially gendered as girls? How do we value different naturally-occurring versus pharmaceutically-adjusted hormone levels between younger and older women, and those with endocrine issues? How does cancer-initiated hysterectomy differ from removal of the uterus during gender reassignment surgery when both procedures are practically identical? These questions point to contradictions embedded in essentialist assumptions regarding gender that underlie questions about the authenticity of trans men's experiences.

Krista Scott-Dixon, a Canadian Women's Studies scholar, explores in her anthology *Trans/Forming Feminisms* (2006) the relationship between feminism and trans experience, unpacks social constructions within the dominant gender binary, and engages in a critical dialogue about the implications of trans-feminisms. Scott-Dixon highlights the importance of framing 'trans' as "a social and political, rather than a medical and psycho-therapeutic, category" (p. 18). In doing so, she brings to the forefront the subjective experience over that of the medical one. The author contends it is within the latter category that trans people face the greatest amount of stigma due to being non-normatively gendered as opposed to those who experience the gender privilege of "normatively and unambiguously placed within a mainstream gender system" (p. 20). Later, in the Discussion chapter, I will explore how gender privilege may benefit some trans men, particularly those who are 'read' more easily as men than others.

Scanlon (2006) furthers this particular discussion with his elaboration on what he calls biocentrism:

> The privilege of being a person whose assigned sex at birth matches their gender identity throughout their lives...the assumption that people who 'match' in this way are more 'real' and/or more 'normal' than those whose assigned sex at birth is incongruent with their gender identity. (p.88)

Non-trans people run the risk of seeing trans as non-normative and thereby subjugating the behaviours of trans people as abnormal. Thus the review of any present literature requires this critical lens in order to identify such bias and within which we must heed Cole, Denny, Eyler and Samons' (2000) caution about a thoughtful use of language because terms like 'disorder' may predispose a reader toward seeing trans people as deficient or mentally ill. "When resorting to the traditional medical-psychology model, it is difficult to discuss transgendered persons or their issues without using terms that imply or overtly state pathology" (p.163).

I have concerns specifically related to the utility of feminism in the exploration of trans men's identity. I am apprehensive that the inclusion of feminism in a discussion of transmasculine people might perpetuate for some the idea that trans men are essentially women. Regardless of how they may self-identify, they are perceived by some as having experienced the world as girls and women and therefore some part of them will always remain female. But is there an essential subjective experience of being a girl who grows up to be a woman? Is this experience different for those for whom a dissonance between inner/outer gender exists? These are some of the questions I continue to wrestle with as I attempt to frame my own research and praxis.

Feminism, particularly social-constructionist feminism, provides a useful analysis of power and oppression within a patriarchal society. Cole, Denny, Eyler and Samons (2000) describe how this work helps us understand how the organization of gender into a binary contributed to a 'transgender model' that evolved in the early 1990s when notions of multiple, perhaps infinite, sexes re-emerged and the anatomic phenotype 'sex' and psychological phenomenon 'gender' began to decouple. Further, they suggest that as gender roles dissolved, more people began to see themselves as both man and women, neither man nor woman, or as an entirely different gender: "Under this model, the in-between state somewhere between manhood and womanhood...[is] a goal for which to strive, or at least a comfortable place at which to rest" (p.160-161).

Still, Judith Lorber (2005) contends that the transition experience, or what she refers to as the "phenomenon of transgendering" is "meaningless without established gender categories" (p.26). Further, she suggests that it is because of these categories that trans people feel the need to engage in this process and be 'read' as the desired gender for the purpose of operating in daily life rather than subverting the gendered social order. Here I believe she addresses the pragmatism of transition previously described by Scanlon (2006). As Irish academic Myra Hird (2000) suggests: "Let me be clear that my objective is not to highlight the difficulties of 'including' intersexuals and transsexuals as women, but rather to question how *anyone* claims this membership based on the current 'sex/gender' binary." (p.350, original emphasis).

This critical lens allows us to understand more fully the complexities of the trans experience within the broader context of trans peoples' lives. As Scott-Dixon explains (2006):

Focusing on trans people alone as subjects of study does not capture the ways in which even normatively gendered people might support or subvert gender roles and regimes. The privilege of being 'perfectly' gendered is also racialized, classed and shaped by other elements of social location, such as age, ability and sexuality, all of which affect how we perceive our gender, and how others perceive us. (p.18)

Gender identity, like sexual orientation or race, is not the only point of oppression or privilege an individual is going to experience. Also problematic is the assumption that the experiences of one oppression are the same as another. For example, the grouping of trans and queer people into a so-called LGBT community is necessarily problematic in that it suggests that the experiences of LGB people in terms of *sexual* identity are identical to those of trans people and their *gender* identity. As Forshee (2008) explains, "the conflation of sexual orientation and gender identity confuses research on each population's unique needs and perspectives." (p.232) While some trans people also identify as queer, these are different journeys altogether, albeit with some similar social ramifications. Thus the reason queer and trans people have historically come together may not be because they share a similar inner journey, but rather that in 'coming out' we face similar oppression, often at the same time, as Stryker (2008) described.

Life satisfaction, subjective well-being and quality of life

Shin and Johnson (1978) define quality of life as a global

assessment of a person's well-being according to individually chosen criteria (p.478). Examining trans men's experiences through the lens of life satisfaction is a way to remove the limitations imposed by the lenses of mental illness diagnoses. Originally I considered exploring experiences of 'happiness'; unfortunately the term, described by Chekola (1974) as the harmonious interplay of a person's goals and desires, is so commonly and broadly used today that the definitions are too many and too vague. Moreover, I was concerned that the term 'happiness' inferred a necessarily positive subjective experience that I wanted to avoid in this project.

In the literature, life satisfaction falls under the broader psychological construct of subjective well-being. According to Diener (1984), subjective well-being is composed of three elements: first, it is based solely on the inner experience of the individual rather than fact; second, subjective well-being is assessed by considering the presence of positive factors as well as a lack of negative factors; and finally, this assessment is global in nature, meaning that individuals generalize their experience despite potentially feeling that some domains of their lives are sub-optimal. He further states that subjective well-being "stresses pleasant emotional experiences" and their relationship to unpleasant ones (p.547). Diener explains: "This may mean either that the person is experiencing mostly pleasant emotions during this period of life or that the person is predisposed to such emotions, whether or not he or she is currently experiencing them." (p.543) According to Ryff (1989), the realms of life people tend to focus on when assessing their subjective well-being include self-acceptance, positive relations with others, autonomy, environmental mastery, purpose in life, and personal growth.

Similar categories are measured in research focused on quality of life (QOL), an area of inquiry that, according to Newfield, Hart, Dibble and Kohler (2006), uses tools to assess "the level of functioning and perceived well-being in a patient population" (p.1448). Results from Jamison Green's (2009) online survey of trans men's sexual satisfaction found that 87.9% of almost 1,300 respondents reported average or better than average QOL using a single item query. Newfield and colleagues (2006), in their online study of 376 participants, found trans men scored lower than the American national average in the areas of mental health (Vitality, Role Emotional, Mental Health, and Mental Health Summary Score) and for social functioning (reflecting physical and/or emotional impact on social activities) which suggests decreased mental-health related QOL (p.1450). These researchers used a well-replicated QOL questionnaire with a group of participants who were mostly white (89%) with a mean age of 32.6. Last year, Colt Meier and Kara Fitgerald (2009) found similar results in their online survey of 369 FTM using the same QOL tool as Newfield and colleagues; participants were mostly white (76.7%), with an average age of twenty-eight.

THEORETICAL FRAMEWORKS

Models of transgender identity development

Little empirical literature exists about transgender identity development (Maguen, Shipherd & Harris, 2005), however two developmental models and a categorical framework have been proposed to understanding experiences of trans people. In her book *Transgender Emergence: Therapeutic Guidelines for Working With Gender-Variant People and Their Families,* American social worker Arlene Lev (2004) describes the six stages of her model of "transgender emergence," the "developmental process whereby gender-variant people examine themselves and their identity, within a context of compassion and empowerment, and progress to an authentic and functional sex- and gender-identity congruence" (p. xx). Informed by an early version of Aaron Devor's (1997) 14-stage model of trans identity development discussed later, Lev's approach uses a postmodern lens to deconstruct gender, sexual orientation, and the diagnostic categories used to treat transgender people. As Harding and Feldman (2006) stated in their review of the book, the title alone is a "reminder that the experience of sexuality and gender does not occur within a vacuum but within the context of family and community systems and their not always supportive reactions" (p.628).

Developed through many years of counseling her trans clients, Lev's (2004) six stages begin with *Awareness*, wherein individuals recognize a sense of difference as the authentic self emerges. They recognize that they cannot deny a history of cross-gender thoughts and behaviours. The result for many is a state of emergency caused by severe psychological pain.

In the second stage, *Seeking Information and Reaching Out*, people seek out narratives and sometimes theoretical and political materials to inform their internal process, resources that are now much more accessible via the Internet. Individuals reach out and often disclose for the first time to a therapist or group, develop one-on-one relationships, and begin to re-examine personal histories.

In the third stage, *Disclosure to Significant Others*, many will have the desire to reveal themselves to partners, family and friends and yet feel conflicted and frightened at the impact this will have on those they love; avoidance is common, as is fear of discovery of cross-gendered behaviours by intimates.

Upon reaching the fourth stage, *Exploring Identity and Transition*, they are considering labels like 'transgender' and 'transsexual,' exploring gender role performance, the importance of passing[3], and options like testosterone replacement therapy (TRT) and GRS. Lev cautions this is one of the most difficult stages with increased risk for mental health and substance-use issues for those without strong coping skills. During the fifth stage, *Exploration: Transition Issues and Possible Body Modifications,* transgender people are making decisions about Homone Replacement Therapy (HRT) and GRS, often beginning treatment, and beginning to living more regularly as their affirmed gender. While for trans men, the effects of HRT are generally sufficient in order that they can be 'read' or perceived as male, some trans women come to terms with the possibility of always being seen as trans. Generally, with the sixth stage, *Integration and Pride*, trans people have completed desired surgeries and made decisions about living 'out' as trans or more 'stealth[4]' and invisible in their community. They go through a process of synthesis of self and integration of the gender they were socialized as, and that which they currently live.

At first glance these stages do resemble a 'coming out' process and, indeed, Lev borrows from models of gay and lesbian identity formation. For Lev, 'coming out' is about self-disclosure of personal and often stigmatizing information (p.229). These stages do seem to have a teleological end-goal of reaching the sixth stage, though Lev does caution that people may move back and forth and revisit stages. She also states that factors like race and access to financial resources impact the process (p.234).

Aaron Devor (2004), a Canadian sociologist at the University of Victoria, proposes a model of 14 stages of transgender identity development based on many years of extensive research, interviews, and both personal and professional interactions with trans people. According to Devor two concepts are foundational to all identity formation: witnessing and mirroring. Witnessing refers to the desire

[3] Passing – the degree to which a person is regarded as a member of the gender with which they physically present
[4] Stealth – describes a person who is read as their affirmed gender at all times and may live apart from those who knew their gender history

we have to be seen by others as we see ourselves. Mirroring involves seeing oneself in the eyes of someone who is similar, a person with an insider perspective on the group with which we identity (Devor, 2004). The 14 progressive stages are:

1) abiding anxiety;

2) identity confusion about originally assigned gender and sex;

3) identity comparisons about originally assigned gender and sex;

4) discovery of transsexualism and transgenderism;

5) identity confusion about transsexualism and transgenderism;

6) identity comparisons about transsexualism and transgenderism;

7) tolerance of transsexual and transgender identity;

8) delay before acceptance of transsexual and transgender identity;

9) acceptance of transsexual and transgender identity;

10) delay before transition;

11) transition;

12) acceptance of post-transition gender and sex identities;

13) integration; and

14) pride.

Although transition is an individualized process, according to Devor (2004) the narratives of identity formation emanating from the above 14 stages have common elements. Many transsexuals experience discomfort at early stages of identity formation in reaction to the dichotomous gender roles imposed in Western society. Some grow increasingly agitated in response to family and friends' discouragement of non-normative gender behaviour and then seek out groups that come closer to matching their internal sense of gender, often among lesbian women and gay men. Some have an epiphany on discovering transsexualism and meeting people within transgender communities. Online resources may inform a tentative self-assessment of transgender identity and a reflection on the possible impacts on self and others. After meeting a trans person for the first time some will quickly self-identify as transsexual, while others take more time; encouragement and support are vital at this stage and throughout the process, as are having people with whom, and places where, they can be open about their experiences. Lack of support, resources and concerns about acceptance may fuel indecision.

Devor (2004) goes on to state that individuals experience a wide range of emotions from elation and relief to sadness at losing part of their life-long identity. Transition is complete for some when they are witnessed within their social networks and communities as the gender to which they wish to transition, while others may choose HRT and GRS. Once transitioned, living as the affirmed gender may feel surreal for a time. Most transsexual people eventually find themselves "seamlessly integrated into society at large" (Devor, 2004, p. 17) and with decreased need for being witnessed. Comfortable with the lived gender experience, they may develop personal pride and the desire to speak more publicly about their lives and communities.

While Devor cautions that this model does not represent the experience of all transsexuals, for this discussion it is important to clarify that issues of race, class, ability, biological receptivity to testosterone, and health status are all mitigating factors that can have substantial impacts on individuals' experiences of transition. Further, Elijah Adiv Edelman (2009), seemingly viewing the model as a purely progressive process, believes that Devor's final two stages are "antithetical in nature" in that they make "it impossible to both live as stealth and be an advocate for trans issues; stealth is rendered as a particular stage in developmental sequence" (p.168) Devor (2004) states that people can go through the stages in different orders. Maguen, Shipherd and Harris (2005) report anecdotal evidence of the model fitting well in their therapeutic work with transsexual American veterans, particularly as evidence of the motivation for some enlisting as an act of performing a gender-stereotyped behaviour. These authors concur with Devor by offering the caveat that "the model is a heuristic for each of the stages a given individual passes through [and that] there are many individual variations in the quest for a cohesive transgender identity" (pp.480-481).

Griffin Hansbury (2005), a trans man and social worker in New York, described from his therapeutic and personal experience three broad categories of transmasculine identity along a spectrum that inform the therapeutic needs of trans men. 'Woodworkers' are the "run-of-the-mill, Joe-six-pack, female-to-male transsexuals" who

identify simply as men and often live under the radar (p.246).
'Transmen' occupy the center of Hansbury's transmasculine spectrum
who acknowledge their past history as female-bodied persons and the
journey of ongoing transition. 'Genderqueers' tend to deny and defy
classification of any particular gender even if their appearance suggests
masculine identity; these folks tend to experience the greatest amount
of stigma. With these categories and the subgroups — transfag, boy-
chick, new man, ungendered — Hansbury brings to the forefront
issues of identity in terms of how individuals relate to one another
along a spectrum of identities. Gayle Salamon (2005) writes:

> Hansbury convincingly argues that transmasculinity can best
> be understood not as fidelity to any single ideal of gendered
> embodiment, or conformity to a singular fantasy of the
> uniformly male body, but rather as a range of masculine bodily
> expressions and feelings. His emendation of the totalizing
> concept of community with the language of the spectrum
> allows masculinity to be understood as a *way* of being (more
> or less masculine) rather than a *kind* of being (transmen versus
> nontransmen), less a fixed ontology of transgenderism and
> more a performative account of transgenderism.
>
> (p.266, original emphasis)

Hansbury is interested in the recognition of a transmasculine
'community' – language he both uses and problematizes – and identity
as it relates to individuals' narrative rather than their behaviours.

These models provide a rough framework that helps those less familiar with trans identity to situate both research and narratives about trans experience within the context of trans lives. The risk of models such as these is that researchers and practitioners may interpret them as a teleological narrative and then assume that all trans people will have the same experience. This risk is still, in my opinion, less than that posed by traditional frameworks for trans healthcare that privilege the medical transition experience and ignore the fundamental psychosocial impacts of transphobia.

Medical & psychiatric etiologies as pseudo-identity models

While trans people and allies were creating new models to understand trans identities, the medical institution had already attempted to describe it from a place of pathology: the *disorder* in Gender Identity Disorder. According to Cole, Denny, Eyler and Samon (2005), physicians and psychiatrists have for decades attempted to understand the origins of transsexualism, some borrowing from Freud's theory of gender as learned behaviour, others using male child victims of surgical accidents whose parents were encouraged to raise them as girls as experiments in nature versus nurture. Scientists looked for explanations within the brain and along the genetic code. By the 1970s clinicians had created a number of categories to describe those who were non-normatively gendered, and yet by the following decade these were already found insufficient:

As more members of the transgender community have come to

> question a system in which there are only two possible
> genders (male and female), the historical categories of
> crossdresser and transsexual have become but two of a
> number of other possible self-identities. (p.151)

According to these authors, as physicians and psychiatrists continued to find discrete categories to label trans people, trans communities blossomed through words and actions, writing books and creating their own organizations without regard to, and perhaps in spite of, the efforts of well-meaning but ill-informed scientists.

A central figure in the history of transsexualism is endocrinologist Harry Benjamin, author of *The Transsexual Phenomenon* (1966), who was a pioneer among medical professionals, and one of the first to speak publicly in support of GRS for transsexuals in the mid-1960s. His statements against psychotherapeutic cures for transsexuals, and encouragement of the medical profession to instead support transsexuals in the gender transition, were groundbreaking for their time (Lev, 2004). What were once the Harry Benjamin International Gender Dysphoria Association *Standards of Care*, first released in 1979, are now the revised *Standards of Care* of WPATH, the World Professional Association for Transgender Health (Meyer, Bockting, Cohen-Kettenis, Coleman, DiCeglie, Devor et al., 2011).

These guidelines are written by, and geared toward, professionals seeking informed recommendations regarding psychiatric, psychological, medical, and surgical management of GID.

In the guidelines, WPATH prescribes the role of mental health providers as those who provide education and psychotherapy, diagnose GID, and conduct assessment or readiness for hormones and surgery. For example, they recommend three months of 'real-life experience' (RLE) in the affirmed gender before prescribing hormones. Another requirement is mental health assessment of transgendered status prior to any surgical procedures, one that places providers and surgeons in a power position as 'gatekeepers' and ostensibly forces trans men people to 'prove' their trans-ness. This assessment ideally incorporates reasonable use of professional judgment that will 'do no harm' when conducting the necessary 'due diligence' with any patient seeking medical treatment, however, the reality remains that this does place mental health professionals in a power position. Treatment guidelines available from the Transgender Health Program at Vancouver Coastal Health (Bockting, Knudsen and Goldberg, 2006) have some of the same limitations while offering useful suggestions for clinicians to mitigate the power imbalance of their relationships with trans patients. They recommend normalizing feelings about the power imbalance, discussing the systemic nature of the assessment process, and remaining transparent about the course of treatment (p.B3). Programs such as Callen-Lorde in New York City recognize the benefit that beginning HRT can have on an individual's mental health and, as a result, have moved toward an *Informed Consent Model* which requires only an assessment of decision-making capacity and the informed consent to take hormones, thus foregoing the 'lived-experience' requirement (Douglass, 2009).

The medical system focuses primarily on gender-reassignment interventions for trans men, and the co-morbidities of GID/GD (Lev, 2004, Raj, 2002; Smit, 2006). Reassignment options for trans men include HRT and gender reassignment surgery (GRS) procedures, although many opt to forego surgical options (Lev, 2004). According to published guidelines from the Endocrine Society (Hembree, Cohen-Kettenis, Delemarre-van de Waal, Gooren, Meyer, Spack, et al., 2009), HRT is typically handled through an intramuscular injection of testosterone, while transdermal and oral forms are also available but more costly. The physical changes caused by testosterone may include growth of facial and body hair, enlargement of the erectile organ (more commonly referred to by trans men as the penis, clitoris or 'clit-dick'), thickening of vocal chords causing the voice to lower, an increase in muscle mass and redistribution of body fat, and male-pattern baldness. To my knowledge, genetic, biological and racial differences in the HRT effects have yet to be studied. Health risks associated with HRT include heart disease, elevated cholesterol, elevated hemocrit and polycythmia, and potential liver damage (especially from oral testosterone). The most common GRS procedures are chest masculinization (commonly referred to as 'top surgery') and hysterectomy and oophorectomy, while less common are genital surgeries such as metoidioplasty, phalloplasty and scrotoplasty (Hembree et al., 2009). In terms of the beneficial effects of testosterone, Newfield and her colleagues (2006) reported from their online survey of 376 FTM that those who had received testosterone had significantly higher QOL score than those who did not.

There are concerns related to mental health and substance use for trans men, though the literature in general about this population is small and contradictory (Lawrence, 2007). Kenagy and Hsieh (2005) report of 69 trans men who participated in HIV-prevention needs assessments conducted in Philadelphia and Chicago in 1997. Data were collected through one-on-one interviews and based on questions developed through focus groups with trans people. They found that 26.2% of participants had previously attempted suicide and, of these, 52.9% (17 respondents) related this action to their gender identity when they answered 'yes' to the question: 'Did you attempt suicide because you are transgendered?'

Clements-Nolle, Marx, Guzman and Katz (2006) reported findings from participatory action research on HIV prevalence conducted in 1997 with transgender communities in San Francisco that may help us understand the state of mental health generally among trans men. Of 586 total participants recruited through trans-identified outreach workers, 123 were trans men. Of these participants, 24 (20%) had a lifetime history of mental-health hospitalization, 39 (32%) had a previous lifetime suicide attempt, and 68 (55%) were depressed based on the Center for Epidemiologic Depression Scale (CES-D).

The mental health literature regarding trans people is highly problematic. As Anne Lawrence (2007) states, the assessment of this literature shows conflicting results wherein some find elevated levels of psychopathology, while others find little or no difference in incidence rates compared to population norms (p.489). Attempts to interpret these reports are made more difficult by the generally small sample sizes of many studies, and by methodological problems such as a lack of standardized psychiatric-assessment tools. The issue I take with Lawrence is that while she recommends bringing a critical lens to the literature, the lens she uses herself is limited to methodological issues and does not capture the essence of trans-affirming feminist perspectives.

The work of Maria Lobato and her colleagues (Lobato, Koff, Manenti, Salvador, da Graça, Petry, et al., 2006) requires just such an analysis. The authors attempt to provide a profile of transsexuals in Brazil by describing only the patients who sought treatment at their university-based gender clinic. This excludes those individuals who might choose to pursue only HRT and do not wish to undertake GRS. The authors state that their "Gender Identity Disorder Program" had seen 138 patients, all of whom were enrolled in the study and, while informed consent was given, no mention was made of how the researchers avoided coercion in terms of access to services. They state in the abstract that 88.4% were "male", thereby disrespectfully describing trans-feminine participants by their natal assigned sex rather than by their affirmed gender. The authors describe transsexualism as a "highly disabling condition," which may be representative of cultural differences in Brazil and therefore true for participants in their particular study; however this is counter to the evidence in Lawrence's (2007) review of the literature, and that done more recently by Peggy Cohen-Kettenis and Friedemann Pfäfflin (2009) who stated that in many, but not all, studies transsexuals "generally function well psychologically in the non-clinical range" (n.p.). Further, the findings of focus groups conducted by Callen-Lorde Health Center in New York showed that participants reacted vehemently against this conceptualization of distress in trans people's experiences (Douglass, 2009).

There do seem to be some issues that Lawrence (2007) states are "plausibly linked to the psychological, social, and economic consequences of living as gender-variant persons in an intolerant society" (p.493), including mental health problems, suicide and self-harm, violence, and risk for HIV infection. The links to the aforementioned issues, according to Cohen-Kettenis and Pfäfflin (2009), include social stigma, difficulties of accessing healthcare and loss of social supports, in addition to the stresses related to subjective experiences of incongruent gender. My interpretation of the Lawrence (2007) and Cohen-Kettenis and Pfäfflin (2009) reviews of the mental health literature suggests that the predominant problems trans men face seem to be socially-determined *DSM-IV-TR* Axis 1 disorders such as depression and anxiety.

There is evidence to suggest that transition-related health interventions such as hormone therapy and gender reassignment surgeries improve mental health outcomes for trans people. The previously mentioned report by Newfield and her colleagues (2006) states that HRT independently predicts higher QOL scores (p<0.01) for trans men. Meier and Fitzgerald (2009), also mentioned previously, found trans men who used HRT had lower scores for depression, anxiety and stress, and increased scores for social support and quality of life. These findings suggest that HRT may play a significant role in the mental health of trans men. Further, van Kestern, Asscheman , Megens and Gooren (1997) studied mortality and morbidity in 293 FTM people at their gender clinic in the Netherlands. Results showed that "cross-gender reassignment treatment, which has been shown to increase the wellbeing of transsexuals, is not associated with an increased mortality rate" (p.341) and further that "cross-sex hormone therapy is acceptably safe" (p.342). When considered together with Meier and Fitzgerald (2009 and Newfield and her colleagues (2006), HRTis a both safe and beneficial option for the mental health and wellness of trans men.

There is concern about the degrees of problematic substance use based on a small number of studies as well as the potential for risk when compared to other marginalized groups. Cole, O'Boyle, Emory and Meyer (1997) found in their retrospective analysis of gender clinic attendees in Texas that 26% of 117 FTM reported lifetime histories of substance-abuse problems. Further, "[i]n virtually all of the cases, subjects describe their substance abuse problems as associated with their gender dysphoria issues" (p.17-18). This sample had a mean age of 30 years, 83% had already begun

HRT and 49% had undergone a surgical treatment (mostly chest surgery), 9% had a history of psychiatric conditions not related to GID or substance abuse, and 21% had attempted suicide. The challenge with a report such as this with a decade and a half of purely historical data is that the reader cannot ascertain whether gender-related therapy, HRT and surgery had any positive impacts and improved the mental health of these individuals.

Dutch findings (1997) found different results. Verschoor and Poortinga (1988), in their seven-year retrospective study of 55 'female transsexuals' seeking treatment at a gender clinic, found only 3.8% had previously abused alcohol or drugs; additionally a third had received undefined psychiatric treatment, and 18.6% had at least one suicide attempt. Interestingly, among a literature that is so highly biased toward the deficits of trans people, this study also reported that 55.8% had satisfying relationships with parents and/or siblings, 48% were in stable relationships, and 74.5% were enrolled in school or stably employed.

Kenagy (2002), reporting separately on the Philadelphia data mentioned above, found that 6% of FTMs reported injecting drugs, an area of potential concern in light of cautions published by the United States Department of Health and Human Services (Substance Abuse and Mental Health Services Administration, 2001) regarding the use of injectable hormones as potentially increasing risk for hepatitis C and for injectable substance abuse relapse. More, the potential for liver damage from ongoing hormone treatment is exacerbated by concurrent drug and alcohol use.

A prominent and yet problematic argument in the literature concerns itself with the comparisons of prevalence figures for mental health problems and substance abuse among trans people and lesbian and gay people. Hughes and Eliason (2002) hypothesize that because trans people experience even greater stigma, violence, and marginalization than do lesbian women and gay men, trans people must also use alcohol and drugs at least at equivalent levels. Lawrence (2007) makes a similarly problematic argument that suggests gay and lesbian people display a comparable gender variance to trans people and thus both groups should experience similar health disparities. Unfortunately this argument is based on the problematic fusing of sexual and gender identity described previously by Forshee (2008).

Whether looking at the conflation of sex and gender in the medical literature, the ongoing pathologizing of trans people, or the non-affirming language, the resulting psychiatrically-defined trans identity can only be described as problematic and unhelpful to trans people. While I acknowledge a certain utility to the mental health literature, I use it cautiously as an indicator of where issues for trans men may exist, while being critical in my analysis of any findings. My own findings described in upcoming chapters challenge or contradict this literature on a number of levels. More useful are the models of identity development created by Devor (2004), Lev (2004) and Hansbury (2005), described previously, that are supported in the data from this study.

PRACTICE IN RELATION TO TRANS ISSUES

Role of the care provider in transgender mental health

Service providers can provide pivotal direct services beyond primary care such as counseling, case management, advocacy, and coordination of care. These services are offered through roles in community mental health settings, acute care in hospitals, and legislated agencies such as child-protective services. Within these settings professionals are also in a position to influence policy and practices that affect persons who have or may be vulnerable to mental health disorders. We can advocate for social change for trans people within trans and non-trans communities.

Sophia Pazos (1999) provides general guidelines for how mental health workers can be allies to our trans clients. We do so by increasing our cultural knowledge of trans communities, using a psycho-education to explain how gender identity disorder may or may not impact mental health and thereby dispel transphobic stereotypes, and generally have an understanding of, and patience for, trans clients who may demonstrate resistance to our interventions due to negative experiences with previous service providers who may have attempted to discourage cross-gender behaviours.

Asking the Right Questions 2: Talking with Clients about Sexual Orientation and Gender Identity in Mental Health, Counselling and Addiction Settings (Angela Barbara, Gloria Chaim, Farzana Doctor, and the Centre for Addictions and Mental Health, 2007) is a helpful guide developed in Toronto together with a day-long training for mental health and addictions treatment practitioners. The authors describe two phases of intervention: a one-page assessment completed by clients to describe their sexual and gender identities, and a set of eight open-ended interview items intended for use during assessment or early in the counseling process as a means of informing case planning. They also provide information about identity-related language, additional probes, and plenty of resources that providers can access. First developed in 2004, the authors evaluated the efficacy of the tool through the post-training feedback forms and telephone interviews. The mental health providers who had been trained to use the guide said it raised their awareness, helped them feel more open and sensitive to sexuality and gender issues, and provided a vocabulary with which to speak to clients (p.2).

The one-page assessment includes four questions. The first asks about current relationship status, the gender of current and previous partners, length of relationship, and the significance of that relationship to the client; numerous gender and sexuality options are available, including a blank. Question two asks the client to identify their sexual orientation, again with a multitude of options, and then asks if the client has any concerns or awkwardness in this area they would like to address. The third question is structured like the second in asking about gender identity, with many options and a query about concerns and awkwardness. The final question asks: "Is your reason for getting help (substance use, mental health concerns) related to any issues around your sexual orientation or gender identity?" The form makes an effective statement to trans and non-trans, queer and non-queer people that the agency or practitioner is aware of and interested in providing service to a diverse clientele. For the healthcare provider, the form provides sufficient information to begin conversations along the sexuality and gender continuums, particularly when clients identify these as areas of concern or discomfort.

The eight interview items are more exploratory in nature, delving into issues that the literature has identified as potential areas of mental health concern. The first seven explore experiences of discrimination, age of first awareness, degree of being 'out' in social and professional realms, community involvement, body image and HIV. The final question asks about the use of substances to cope with the previously mentioned issues, and/or whether the mental health issues presented are similarly related. Each is presented as applicable to both sexual and gender identity, a strategy that is effective in broadly shifting practitioner awareness to these issues. This broadness my also be a limitation in terms of addressing trans-specific issues regarding, for example, the personal impacts of internalized transphobia. To their credit the authors introduce Devor's model of identity development as a model to understand the 'coming out' process of transgender people, although the language suggests 'coming out' and transition are for some people one in the same.

According to Cole, Denny, Eyler and Samons (2000), health care providers can intervene using two particular strategies. First, we can engage with trans clients with regard to preventative medical care, and build understanding that bodies in transition are only as healthy as the care that is taken with them. "It is necessary to take care of a body part for as long as it is a part of your body" (p.167). This means addressing the gamut of health issues and behaviours that affect each of us whether trans or non-trans, from smoking and obesity to fitness and mental wellness. And for trans men specifically it means those who retain breast tissue require mammograms, and those with a cervix and uterus require annual pelvic exams. Our second role is to explore and address with clients their histories of interaction within healthcare settings, particularly for abuse or mistreatment. We can then refer clients to practitioners we know to be both welcoming and trained in transgender health. When these physicians, endocrinologists and surgeons require assessments prior to providing medical interventions, general practitioners and mental health service providers may be called upon to provide assessments. In some regions specific individuals may be identified to provide surgical assessment before health insurance will approve coverage, if any. Cole, Denny, Eyler and Samons (2000), Bockting, Knudson and Goldberg (2006) and Lev (2004) explain these assessments at length and in depth.

In *Counselling and Mental Health Care of Transgender Adults and Loved Ones,* Bockting, Knudson and Goldberg (2006) provide clear clinical guidelines for a thorough mental health assessment of transgender clients including clinical pathways, capacity for decision-making, and generally a more comprehensive discussion of assessment criteria within the WPATH *Standards of Care* (2011). In 'Social and

Medical Advocacy with Transgender People and Loved Ones: Recommendations for BC Clinicians', social worker Catherine White Holman and her colleague Joshua Goldberg (2006) provide a contextual perspective of practice with trans people cultivated from many years of clinical experience. They caution about awareness of literacy levels and cultural diversity when conducting any assessments. Practitioners are likely to encounter new immigrants, refugees, and those requiring support who do not speak English. Potential life-areas of intervention that can impact mental health include financial assistance and housing, health and childcare, and advocacy with regard to housing, employment, or in the change of identification. In some cases we may work with individuals with complex mental health and cognitive concerns, and for whom accessing healthcare can be a difficult task in and of itself.

Lev (2004) identifies three reasons for clients to seek assistance regarding gender issues, the first being those gender variant people seeking medical assessment and referral already described; the other reasons have been far less elucidated in the literature. The second is familial or relationship issues that may require additional support to partners and family members (p.204). Lev offers a model of Family Emergence with four stages: Stage 1, *Discovery and Disclosure*, finds individuals reacting to their transgender loved one with feelings of shock, confusion and betrayal; Stage 2, *Turmoil*, finds family members in chaos and stress as they struggle to accept gender variance; Stage 3, *Negotiation*, has family recognizing the gender issues will not dissipate and reaching compromise about how the gender expression can be realized within the family unit; and Stage 4, *Finding Balance*, is respite from the turmoil after negotiation and coming to terms with the now-public secret that was transgenderism.

Lev's third reason for clients to seek help is to address gender-related distress. She argues that the fear trans people have for transgressing normative gender behaviours, and the long-term performance of a false self may actually cause mental health issues (p.196). Lev states:

> The high incidence of mental illness among transgendered people noted in the literature might be better understood as reactive symptomology and posttraumatic sequalae. It is literally *crazy-making* to live a false self. (p.196, original emphasis)

Lev believes that these illnesses might actually be expressions of deep-seated trauma. This approach releases transgenderism and GID/GD as expressions of mental health symptoms and substitutes these with an etiological view of Post-Traumatic Stress Disorder (PTSD), another *DSM* diagnosis that is familiar to practitioners, without the burden of the gender-related stigma. The key, if in fact the foundations of transgender mental health are based in PTSD, is for service providers to explore these issues with their trans clients. I offer an assessment tool in chapter 6 to assist providers to do just that.

Using a strengths-based approach to research

In order to achieve an understanding of individuals' lives, I use a strengths-based model commonly used in community mental health practice as a research lens. As Saleebey (1996) explains:

> The strengths perspective demands a different way of looking at individuals, families, and communities. All must be seen in the light of their capacities, talents, competencies, possibilities, visions, values, and hopes, however dashed and distorted these may have become through circumstance, oppression, and trauma. The strengths approach requires an accounting of what people know and what they can do, however inchoate that may sometimes seem. It requires composing a roster of resources existing within and around the individual, family, or community. (p.297)

This shift in thinking is away from a problem-solving or pathology approach that situates the service provider in the role of expert to one where the health provider is another resource to whom the true experts – our clients – can turn to assist in achieving their self-identified needs. This is not to dismiss the existence of 'presenting problems', the issues that first bring them to our offices. Once client and provider have clarified the issues at hand, Graybeal (2004) recommends they explore the personal, social and community resources the client possesses that could potentially help address the problem. What realistic options does the client see as available? What possible directions are reasonable? When has the presenting problem been less problematic, what was different at that time, and what can the client draw from that experience? And what does the client see as potential solutions?

Saleebey (1996) outlines some of the common critiques of a strengths-based method of practice: it is a guise for 'positive thinking', merely reframes misery, ignores reality, or is naïve. However, rather than a superficial reframe of client problems, the strengths-based approach is one that requires skilled practitioners who seek to meet their ethical obligation to be client-directed in all aspects of their practice. The approach requires us to capitalize on clients' capacities and demonstrated abilities in order to move forward. To do so requires the use of counseling and communications skills to get to the core of client needs and values. We communicate the reality of the challenge, and then help clients develop strategies to work through these. As Cousin (1989) suggests, "one should not deny the verdict (diagnosis or assessment) but should defy the sentence" (cited in Saleebey, 1996, p.303). The answers are found in the stories clients share about their lives and, thus, this model is an effective complement to a narrative research approach, one that elicits from participants stories and then uses these as data for analysis.

This book falls within an evolving movement of researchers, advocates and policymakers who use a wide array of strengths-based approaches. Maton (2004) asserts these groups share a common world-view that seeks to shift away from the deficits-based methods toward explorations of resilience, health promotion, school reform and community development (p.3). Important to this study of trans men are the authors' suggestions that this approach can help to understand healthy development and the role of resilience; empower those lacking power while strengthening environments; and promote individual development, quality of life and self-advocacy (p.4).

We often say that we only want the best for one another. Parents say they just want their children to be happy. A strengths-based assessment provides a broader context in terms of abilities and capacities within which we can learn what's working and what's not. If we do want what is best for others then I think we are interested in wellness and in physical and mental health that are sufficient to support satisfied lives for trans men. How to achieve this is still not well understood, as indicated by the enormous gaps in the present health and mental health literatures described previously. It is my belief that, by highlighting the strengths inherent within the stories of generally-satisfied trans men, we can begin to fill this gap.

APPLICATION OF THEORY, RESEARCH AND PRACTICE

Feminist theory assists in the identification of sites of power and resistance between the institutions that have historically provided healthcare and the various oppressed groups; as yet this tension has only been described in a limited way in terms of trans men. Narrative research, which I discuss in more detail in the Methodology (see Appendices), provides an avenue to elicit from participants the stories of their experiences in the everyday world, while honouring agency and subjectivity (Mishler, 1986). By drawing out stories from trans men about how they understand the world, I can identify and expose how their lives intersect with the hegemonic establishment. The subjective well-being framework explains how any person might assess their own well-being (Diener, 1984; Ryff, 1989), but to date this approach has not been applied to the lives of trans men, nor has it been used, to my knowledge, as a gauge for confirming the life satisfaction of a particular group.

Transgender identity developmental models, such as those proposed by Devor (2004) and Lev (2004), provide a rough framework that helps those less familiar with trans identity to situate both research and narratives about trans experience within the context of trans lives, but have yet to be applied as a method of contextualizing the dominant and medicalized literature on mental health and GID/GD among trans people. As discussed, these developmental frameworks highlight gaps in the medical discourse on transgenderism that focuses on a narrow range of identity-development stages, specifically from the time an individual is exploring resources until they undergo medical interventions. The range of stages encompassed by the medical discourse correspond roughly with Lev's (2004) 'seeking information and reaching out' through to 'integration: acceptance and post-transition issues' (Stages 2 to 5), and with Devor's 'discovery of transsexualism and transgenderism' through to 'transition (Stages 4 to 11). Thus, due to the dominance of the medicalized model in the existing trans literature, we know little about the experiences of those who are early in their consideration of gender and those who have completed transition and have developed their post-transition identity.

The Standards of Care and other frameworks for praxis direct health providers toward treatment that privileges the medical transition experience. These lack the capacity to explore foundational psychological impacts that are a result of gender-related stigma. Lev (2004) hones in on key therapeutic issues, and suggests trauma may be at the root of disordered behaviour. What is still lacking are practical therapeutic tools to unearth those traumatic experiences that may impact the mental health and wellness of trans clients, and an understanding of how those experiences affect the lives of trans people who are not mentally ill. An assessment tool is needed, one that can guide the dialogue between client and provider to understand the impacts of these experiences.

By exploring the subjective experiences of well being through a critical, trans-feminist lens, I aim to counter the dominant, pathologizing discourse. I wondered, what can be learned from the stories of trans men about their mental health and wellness? Further, I endeavoured to understand in which realms of trans men's lives satisfaction is important and/or significant. These are the questions I followed through this research, and that inform the development of an assessment tool for use by health to address transition-related mental health issues.

3 | STORIES OF TRANS MEN

Four themes emerged from the stories men shared about their lives. In the first, I share some of the ways in which they demonstrated how their efforts at managing early transition demonstrated self-efficacy, a key factor in a satisfying transition experience. Next, I discuss how hearing positive stories from previously-transitioned trans men offered hope during transition. Then I describe how personal supports and resources directly impacted the 'success' of transition. Finally, I show how these trans men charted their own courses to satisfaction.

The importance of transition in the lives of trans men

Transition experience was significant for the men I spoke with and, within this, several issues relating to early transition such as realizing they are trans, connecting with other trans people, 'passing' or being 'read' as a man and how this experience can be different for those with other marginalized identities.

The guys each described in their own way how they first self-acknowledged being trans. Half of them indicated they were aware of a gender disharmony or of being male since childhood or youth, while just as many others came to this realization in their early to mid-twenties. While there was no consistency among the guys about the length or context of their early gender ruminations, each did speak of a moment or epiphany when they recognized a desire for exploring gender and this was the impetus for beginning their transition journey. As Jimmy (a pseudonym, as are all names included here) explained:

> If this is my truth, if this is what I lay in bed on a Saturday morning fantasizing about doing if I won the lottery, then what's really stopping me from doing it? And yeah, I haven't looked back.

Here he describes a standard with which an individual might measure their desire for an important decision in life. This is a scene most people can relate to, inviting us to consider what we might dream for ourselves if afforded that same space to daydream. For Jimmy the persistent truth remained the same in that he wanted to transition and he used this time to reflect on and affirm his decision to do so. Based on the smile on his face as he spoke these words, he was clearly happy he followed though with his decision.

Arthur spoke differently about his gender epiphany and decision to transition:

> And so I was a girl for a while and I was okay being that. There wasn't any problem but I knew there was something else for

me to explore, right. So when I was 33, I just kind of thought: "Well, okay, I think I'm done being a girl. Let's go be something else." And that's just what I did. It wasn't some horrible traumatic thing from the past with gender dysphoria. It just was what it was: I always wanted to be a boy, sure.

[And] I didn't kind of give myself a hard time about it either. This story counters the dominant medical narrative that there must be long-term struggle or anxiety about gender. Arthur normalizes the experience as just another option to be considered and goal to be achieved. Clearly we must not make any assumptions about how these trans men first came to recognize their trans-ness.

In the early stages of transition, many of the men sought out support groups in order to meet others with similar revelations, which arguably put them in a privileged position over others who did not have similar access. One man referred to a popular Vancouver support group as "a weekly or a monthly bitch session" where attendees spoke only about what was hard in their lives and the issues with which they were struggling. What became clear was that these men were not averse to the people attending the groups, but rather to the negative tone and content of discussions there. Troy described his experience very clearly: "I ended up hating going to the group later on because of the negativity." He continued attending a support group for trans men for a number of months until he finally stopped. He, like many others, described his frustration at hearing what was not working for support group attendees, and rarely hearing any solutions.

Another fellow, Abraham, said:

> I feel like if there had been other kinds of [stories] out there.
> Not to say that talking about the tough stuff isn't important to
> you. I think that's super critical, right? And I like being able to
> share that with other folks. But also having other examples...a
> more broad range of experiences that you're going to go
> through, right? Rather than just, "oh my God, this is all doom
> and it's hell," and you know...how to live in a more positive
> way and hearing more stories of guys going through this kind
> of stuff and living well and treating themselves well.

Abraham was seeking stories other than those shared at the group.
While he saw value in having a venue for trans men to express their
frustrations, he also wanted to hear a broader range of stories from
trans men who were doing well and had utilized effective strategies
that could be helpful to other group members. The dominance of
negative stories in the accounts of support groups identifies one of the
primary challenges they were encountering. As practitioners who refer
people to support groups, we hope that our clients will get positive
support rather than 'horror stories', however expressing the
difficulties seems to be part of the process. For those sharing their
challenges it may be therapeutic, while for those hearing them it may
be the impetus they need to seek out different stories.

Problems were not limited to support groups. Ming recounted
his interpretation of the troublesome perspective on transition that
the psychiatrists shared during an assessment:

Right from the beginning when I chose to go and see the two shrinks [laughs]. They tell you whether or not they think that you are [trans] based on their analysis. I was aware, I'm [a person]of colour, right, and here are two people who are white telling me: 'Oh alright, so what's going to happen is you're going to get all hairy and smell a certain way and you're gonna get really big." And I said to him, 'I'm gonna become a guy. I'm not going to become a white guy.' I got at that moment that the model on which transitioning was all based was on white. I went, 'Ah okay, this is a whole world that doesn't even relate to me. So I'm just going to go out and create my own path.'

Ming was conscious that the assessment by the psychiatrist was external to him and that there existed a power differential. At the same time he was aware of his own Other-ness in this situation; he was a person of color and the psychiatrists were white. They did not see differences in the effects of testosterone on people of color that this man had already considered. He was aware of his own biology and genetic predisposition and recognized that, as an Asian man, he was neither likely to grow substantial facial and body hair nor gain a great amount of size. He would become a man, but not in the image of a white man. It was struggles like this one to overcome a particular hurdle that allowed these men to demonstrate the resilience they needed to proceed with their transition plans.

There was an awareness that they brought to their early transition where, in some cases, they were able to identify the lack of pragmatic strategies that would be helpful in transition. In other cases they just knew something was missing and that the stories they were hearing were only focused on what was not working. Their lives were not miserable, and they did not want others at the group to negatively affect their state-of-mind.

Julian brought an insightful analysis to the utility of the negative and positive stories:

> I'm looking for positive stuff but I also acknowledge that there is a history there where we, as a group of [trans] people, have had to rely on those negative stories to get the care that we require.

Julian was aware of the political contexts within and through which trans men have moved and participated in order to access health care. In many cases the guys spoke of exaggerating their experiences in an effort to subvert the system and get their needs met. There was recognition of the dependence trans men have on the health care system and the relationship each person has with that system.

These men each described themselves as being post-transition, each using a unique subjective assessment. As post-transition trans men, they brought hindsight to their recollection of their experiences in early transition. A common topic they described was 'passing' or being 'read' as a man in social interactions, which in my experience is a highly charged concept within trans communities due to interpretations of inauthenticity. 'Passing' was explored by the guys in a number of ways and contexts. One shared:

> I mean some of [my satisfaction] has to do obviously with 'passing,' um, like I mentioned in the group. Like I don't feel this, like, angst every time I leave my house because someone's going to beat the shit out of me 'cause they can't tell what's going on with me.

This fellow spoke clearly to the social anxiety trans men experience as a result of being perceived as gender variant while in public and how the resulting confusion is for some people sufficient impetus to act out violently. In terms of personal well-being, he believed 'passing' helped to lower his anxiety. Others shared similar concerns.

Some guys were aware of differences between transmasculine and transfeminine experiences and that, in terms of passing, those on the transfeminine spectrum often have a much more difficult time. As the men embarked on their transitions and particularly when they began TRT, they had a great deal of anxiety going out into the world with a more gender ambiguous appearance. One stated:

> It can be totally exhausting just being you. It can be emotionally overwhelming just walking in society. But since I have a beard I [only] get 'she' occasionally from the bus driver.

As this man demonstrates, it is in everyday exchanges that non-normative gender presentation can be stressful. This anxiety remains despite knowledge that the masculinizing effects of hormones, particularly testosterone, generally happen more quickly for trans men than trans women – over weeks and months rather than years – and that they would likely not require additional surgeries to 'pass' as long as their breast are of a size that can be concealed. They feared that an androgynous face and a higher-pitched voice would reveal them as trans and thus they practiced masculine manners of walking and moving. One man shared:

> I didn't pass as quickly as most people I know do. I didn't change my mannerisms a lot. I still talk with my hands a lot and that sort of thing... There's lots of these little things that in the beginning [other trans men] tell you you have to do to pass.

Additionally, the significance of growing facial hair as an unambiguous marker of masculinity cannot be overstated in terms of subjective well-being; this epiphany was consistent among the six guys who were able to do so and the two who were not because of genetic or biological factors.

Appearing as a man is only one level of 'passing,' while having supporting documentation of a masculine identity was another important component, although not always easy to access depending on how effectively individuals could 'pass' in social contexts. This challenge is highlighted in this brief dialogue from one of our large group discussions:

> *Speaker 1:* My driver's license had expired and I remember going down to the driver's license bureau and, I always got mistaken for being a guy. It's like ever since I was knee high to a grasshopper. I went in and thought, 'I wonder if I can get them to change the gender of my driver's license without proving that I'm a guy.' And so I remember going up to the

counter and said, 'Oh, by the way, they made a mistake on my driver's license. They put an 'F' on and I never changed it because it's just, like, a hassle. But now that's it expired, can you...?' She's like, 'Oh my god, I'm so sorry. I'll fix that.' And all of a sudden I had a driver's license.

Speaker 2: They didn't want to do that to me. They're, like, 'No, you need to show me another piece of ID.'

The first speaker talked about having had a masculine appearance even as a young person and he used this to his advantage in this powerful act of transgression. Later in the discussion he made it clear he was aware of the social investment in a gender binary as he spoke with the agent at the licensing office. Someone with a gender-neutral name like he had, and who presented so unambiguously as male could only be that sex and therefore the categorization as female on the driver's license must be a clerical error. For the licensing office agent, there was perhaps no space for gender alternatives in that exchange. Also interesting is how he stated at the end that suddenly he had a driver's license when clearly he had had one previously; this was a five-year renewal that required a new photograph and the issue of a new license card. What was different for this speaker was that now his driver's license held new meaning and was useful for supporting his affirmed gender in the world. No longer did it have attached to it the low-grade anxiety that might come along with knowing that his gender could be questioned by any police officer pulling him over for speeding or a broken tail light.

The second speaker had a different experience when he renewed his driver's license. The clerk was unwilling to change the gender without seeing an additional piece of identification. He believed that this was purely a policy-based, bureaucratic decision on behalf of the agent, however, the importance of 'passing' as male socially cannot be ruled out. He did not have the same traditional masculine markers as did some of the others. While they sported beards and revealed chest hair above their shirts, this man's youthful, hairless presentation may have raised red flags for the licensing clerk, and perhaps the clerk had other knowledge or experiences that influenced the decision. Regardless, there was a disparity in the experiences that these trans men had depending on how effectively they were able to 'pass' as male in society. Related to this disparity there reside varying levels of social anxiety, which, as previously stated, are connected to concerns for personal safety.

Overall, there were a number of small issues raised by these men in regard to this significant experience they call "transition." From the personal epiphany of recognition, through support group meetings and mental health appointments, to the perceptions of the outside world, these men were challenged and ultimately demonstrated their capacities for self-efficacy.

Positive stories from other trans men offer hope

At our first group meeting, one man reflected on the personal impact of meeting a groups of trans men who had a different story to share from what he had heard previously: "I kind of knew, even hearing my first positive story, that there was hope and I was going to get there." What this quote revealed is that when this fellow heard that first story he already had a sense of hope; this story was more of a confirmation. He said, "I kind of knew," suggesting that this was an ongoing feeling that he had been having. Clearly he had been not just *looking* for positive stories, but had made a unilateral categorization of previously-heard stories as negative and unhelpful. With the benefit of hindsight from the position of a post-transition trans man, he was able to define that first positive story and use it for comparison to the negative stories he had heard from peers and healthcare providers. The impetus, however, that came from that story was that he could continue on and complete his transition. He might have the same degree of success as was described in that first positive story he had heard.

Numerous accounts shared by the guys confirmed that negative stories presented by peers and healthcare providers were pervasive and unhelpful. The negative stories that the guys heard described a particular way of going about transition that was fraught with barriers and challenges. On reflection, one man offered this advice: "I just want some positive [stories]. I want people to know that you don't have to have this script. You don't have to do it this way to be happy, you know." He referred to a "script" that a person can choose to follow, and thus infers both alternative scripts and the agency of the individual to select among them. He described a prescribed path that trans men are expected to follow and, as I will discuss later, this path privileges the medical experience of transition over the individual one. He needed positive stories to counter the negative ones that are so insidious in trans communities his advice for others, as much as for his younger self when he was still in his transition, was that trans men might find happiness along alternative paths. Another fellow also spoke about countering the dominant stories about trans men in transition when he said:

> Trans people right now are the sexy topic. And the sexy topic seems to be, you know, they're alcoholics, they're prostitutes, drug addicts, they're this, they're that.

This man was aware of the community-level impact when negative stories about trans people become the "sexy topic", as well as the broader societal impact of those stories. These stories feed larger narratives about trans men and trans people that perpetuate the ongoing pathologization of these communities.

The guys did not deny the existence of challenges, nor did they deny the merit of hearing about the challenges. What they wanted to be different was to balance the challenges with stories from those who had found their way through them.

> There were a few more people, sort of the more senior people in the community. I found that they didn't actually share as much. They'd answer sort of technical questions, you know. "Who's a good doctor for this?" You know, "I need to find a psychologist." You know, "Is there anything I can do about my

acne?" All these sorts of technical, practical questions. They were more than happy to answer that. But I didn't get a lot of, 'This is my life and this is where it rocks' kind of stuff from people. And I looked for it.

This man clearly saw a hierarchy within the community. The individuals whom he referred to as "senior people" seemed to be those who had progressed further along in their transitions. He had expectations about what information these individuals would provide and they were not meeting those expectations. He talked about them as responding to more mundane questions but, similarly to individuals described here, these "senior people" in the community were reluctant to talk about what worked well in their lives. What he really wanted to hear was some "This is my life and this is where it rocks" stories. This fellow went on to reflect on his awareness of these senior people, their reluctance to share, and talked about his own experience:

> I'm overwhelmingly happy with my life, but I certainly am not sharing that with anybody who is beginning off in transition. I don't know. I wish there was a way I could do that.

Here I heard the first hint of guilt from the guys, a consistent theme in the large group meetings and individual interviews. They identified how content they were in their lives and saw themselves, much like those "senior people", unwilling to share their positive stories. When this fellow said he wished there were a way he could share his stories, it was not for lack of a venue: he knew the whereabouts of the support groups because he had previously attended them. These men saw value in hearing positive stories in that these were in most cases the impetus for getting on with their own journeys. I often asked how they might let their stories be known by other trans men and they commonly responded that they just did not know how, and that they hoped I might be able to do so with this research project.

Personal supports & resources impact transition 'success'

The men in this project identified a number of social supports that were important to them during transition. One spoke about how the eccentricity, issues and personalities *within* his family actually lessened the anxiety that he felt *from* his family.

> My family is just really weird. Everyone's got some odd thing but nobody cares. You know, like nobody really cares. My family is whatever, just be yourself, you know. And that's a good thing. I think, uh, yeah, that's a good thing. Like I always think my friends are the "be all end all". They are so not. It's my family. It always goes back to my family.

This fellow explained during his one-on-one interview that his family situation was quite complicated due to a history of eccentric family dynamics. Ultimately, all of the interpersonal complication raised the bar for this family in terms of what might create tension. Within the context of this particular family, exploration of gender and transitioning was not particularly unsettling.

Personal support came in many other forms. For one man, support came from a best friend and confidant, someone with whom he attended support groups until they realized that they heard nothing there but negative stories; in response they formed their own support group of two. Another fellow talked about the value of his close relationship with his mother and father. Three others spoke about the role strangers had played when they began their transition experience, be it the voice at the other end of a telephone support line or the individual who answered emails through websites. For another it was a trans neighbour who invited him into his social circle of neighborhood trans men and allies.

In terms of resources, the guys spoke of using personal resources like education and knowledge of the healthcare system to navigate through the hoops service providers offered. They talked about utilizing the resources and the relationships they had with service providers in order to get what they wanted. By far the greatest resource that these men accessed was the ability to foreground transition as the primary focus in their lives. One explained:

> Within the first two years I'd sort of wrapped up all the medical stuff, which a lot of people can't. In the community, the people that I have been talking to, that has not been true for them. And so, part of the reason I don't want to go to a group and talk about how awesome my life is because I made some decisions and sacrifices and I had some opportunities that some people don't have. I decided that this is, this is it. This is the most important thing to me right now so I'm just going to do it. And, um, I have the financial means to do that.

> I will be paying it off for the next 15 years but [laughs], I made
> a financial decision that some people aren't able to make.

At first glance what stood out from this quote was the fact that he had the financial resources to be able to afford to not wait for the provincial health insurance plan to pay for the surgery. When the fellow said that this was the most important thing in his life at the time he described not only his desire, but also his ability to make transition the focus of his life for that period of time. He was not restricted by other activities or responsibilities in such a way that he could not do this. As he said, he made sacrifices in other parts of his life so that he could focus primarily on his transition. The men I spoke with sacrificed jobs, ended relationships, and made space in their lives to focus on transition. They had the capacity to identify a goal and understand the potential barriers and challenges to meeting that goal.

Trans men chart their own course to satisfaction

These men each found their own way to work with, operate through, and sometimes against, service providers in order to access the health-care that they wanted. The guys were familiar with the *Standards of Care* and either worked with them or around them. Sometimes even their providers bypassed these. One fellow had a very fortunate experience with his health-care provider,

> I was blessed with a really supportive and accepting doctor. I
> didn't have to find one. He was already there. He listened to
> me. I'd ask him for a referral to a doctor in another city and

he'd write it ...without question. And we had a discussion about what it is that I was doing and where I wanted to go with it and how fast I wanted to go. That opened up a lot of opportunities for me. I didn't have to stick through some sort of arbitrary system of deadlines. With the exception of two, healthcare providers that I dealt with in my entire transition process were really supportive. They'd say things like "Sounds like you've really thought about this. Okay let's just do this."

This man found a physician who was clearly patient-centered and was willing to provide whatever support he needed including a referral to a trans specialist in another city who the the fellow knew would respond more favourably. This was the exception, not the rule, for the guys I spoke with. This man went on to say that he recognized the difference and that others were sharing very different stories.

Some of the stories I've heard from other people about how they were told they weren't trans enough or that they weren't male enough or that they hadn't waited long enough. As if waiting somehow makes it more valid. That's again part of the reason why I stopped playing in the community, because there were all these stories about that. I would get so frustrated. "Why are you putting up with that?" You know, "Why don't you just make a decision about what it is that's going to make you happy and what it is that's going to move you forward in your life and do it." Um, which is sort of a decision I came to on my own.

What emerged from this man's narrative was some recognition of his own frustration at watching others who were not able to pay as much attention their transition and choose transition in the same way that he had. He expected everyone to have the capacity to just make a decision and follow through with it, but in reality that is not the case. There are numerous barriers and challenges that individuals confront in trying to follow through with their hopes and dreams. Also we get a sense of why this fellow, like many others I spoke with, stopped participating in the trans community. They shared a degree of frustration with fellow community members, perhaps fueled by guilt, an issue discussed later in this chapter.

This man had strong opinions about the health-care system, the process that people had to go through, and some of the questions that health-care providers would ask: "I didn't have to go through the bullshit process that lots of people had to go through when they're seeing other surgeons: 'Oh, you're too young. Are you sure you don't want to have kids?'" To answer this hypothetical question, the fellow responded emphatically: "Out of my vagina!? No!" and laughed heartily with the other men in the group. This individual, as did others, recognized the gatekeeper status and a particular mentality that many health-care providers have when dealing with trans people. The language and tone used by healthcare professionals has often been patronizing and suggests that trans men would not know what is best for them. Such physicians seemed more interested in preserving the sanctity of reproductive capacity than honoring the subjective gender-based decisions that trans men are making. These men may not have recognized the ethical responsibilities that professionals have regarding conduct of medical procedures, but accounts like this suggests that their physicians' behaviour and language left some feeling disrespected and with the need to protect themselves.

Another fellow also recognized the challenges of the health-care system for treating trans men. He was concerned for his own mental health and ability to endure that system:

> I knew I didn't have the resilience [laughs] to wait as long as some of those other guys. And I wanted to be one of those [more senior guys] so badly. I knew it was going to get pretty bad if I didn't do something. So it was the desire to not want to be on those darn waiting lists.

For this man it was his understanding of the challenges of maneuvering that system that was in part the impetus for mobilizing himself and increasing his own self-efficacy in order to get his needs met.

Another fellow explained having a self-perception that was quite different to other trans people in terms of social locations:

> Being queer, not binding, being a gimp, not having a job, not wanting bottom surgery, like all this different kind of stuff. It was just a constant battle. And that story kept coming up. I didn't tell the same story. It just wasn't, I didn't, I haven't always felt like a boy. I didn't always want to be a man. I don't want certain kinds of [surgery]. So the idea of challenging those

[negative stories] or –not challenging, that's a bit dramatic, but adding to what those possible stories can be – is sort of what I see this kind of [book] doing. Like adding, like [transition]'s not all about doom and gloom. There's actually some really amazing stuff that comes out of [transition].

This individual had no lifetime of GID/GD, which went contrary to physicians' expectations and the dominant story about trans people's experiences. They self-reported as feeling 'Othered' by trans men in terms of sexuality, presentation, ability, employment and desire for gender reassignment surgery. As with all of the guys, there was an awareness that the dominant model of transition did not match their subjective experience.

In a number of cases the guys talked about actually enjoying their transition experience, an idea that is so far away from that negative story. During a large group session, two of the guys shared an interesting exchange. The first spoke about the journals he had kept for much of his life and, when he went back to look at his entries from the time he began his transition, he saw that he set the specific intent to enjoy his transition experience.

> *Speaker 1:* And I felt like some sort of freak for having enj-, I have enjoyed it. I have enjoyed every moment of it. You know, some moments, the post-op pain and that, not so much. Six days of constipation after my hysterectomy, wasn't enjoying that. Oh I had a brutal, brutal time... I was doped up and in pain, puking. But I was always looking at the positive. It was

the first time in my entire life – well not entire but pretty much since I was about 12 or 13 – that I wasn't, like, in pain, in that [pelvic] region of my body.

Speaker 2: It's amazing the smile you can have on your face when you're puking and you're in the worst pain in your life but it's the happiest moment of your life waking up from surgery.

Through the haze of physical discomfort and pain medication these men stated they were still able to connect with the joy of the journey they were on. Certainly the first speaker was thrilled that he was never going to have menstrual pain again but, more than the embodied experience, his tone suggested to me that another kind of pain was reduced, specifically the one that comes with experiencing a gender-conflicted body process. When an individual experiences himself as a man but continues to have body processes that are inconsistent with his perceived gender, that causes another kind of emotional and, perhaps, psychic pain. I can only imagine what the health-care providers who were observing this man must have thought seeing smiles and joy in the eyes of someone who was in such a painful physical situation; the contrast of these must have been quite a sight to see.

4 | GOING DEEPER

Three individuals' stories stood out as examples of some of the broader narratives described in the previous section. In the first, Ed shares the experience of first taking his shirt off post-chest surgery, providing some insight into how he made meaning of his great life. In the second, Kaleb talks about meeting some of those more senior trans men, and the impact these meetings had on his transition. Lastly, Eric speaks about how he used a little plastic egg to help him through a particularly difficult period in his transition. Their stories are examples of, or contrasts to, the narrative themes shared in the previous chapter.

ED'S STORY
"I was like, 'Yeah, who's the man!'"

When asked, Ed said he identifies as a man, a person who finished his transition eight years ago and thus is no longer trans per se. This was not necessarily the case for other men I spoke with but was one way of being that Ed chose for himself. When he first contacted me by email he wrote: "I feel as though my life has been hugely successful and satisfying for me. I am very positive and happy to be where I am now." I chose to write about Ed's story because his story shared both commonalities and differences with the others in fairly equal measure. In terms of the experiences of trans men I heard, Ed's story seems to be situated in the centre: a fairly typical, middle-class transmasculine experience.

What follows is an account shared by Ed toward the end of his individual interview. He recounted the definitive summer story of a guy taking his shirt off in the heat of the day.

I remember the first day I sort of took my shirt off in public. I was out in [a rural area outside of Vancouver] and it was a beautiful hot sunny day. And I was [thinking] "Nobody here knows me." I'm walking along and it's just like so hot and I knew I could take my shirt off. I was looking around, thinking about it and feeling a little nervous about it. And I thought, "What the hell?" And I took my shirt off and it was just, like, "Oh my god. This feels so great." And about five minutes later, this car full of girls drove by and they all started whistling and yelling at me. It was perfect. It was like, "Yeah, who's the man?!" And I totally had this little ego moment and I felt so excited. It's like I, I chest-passed, I've taken off my shirt. I've got scars on my chest and they're relatively fresh at that point. This car full of girls just drove right past me whistling and waving and screaming at me...I love it. It's the best thing ever [laughs].

Ed set the scene perfectly: a hot summer's day, a revealing of the male torso, a car filled with flirtatious 'hot babes.' Reminiscent for me of Brad Pitt in *Thelma & Louise,* this was like a teenage boy's coming-of-age where he had a desire to be noticed as a man and admired for the body that he had created for himself. In this instance, when Ed marveled that he "chest-passed" it was like a milestone in his 'trans adolescence.' As much as Ed was comfortable within himself this story revealed through the taking off of his shirt a newfound comfort with his body, an integration of body and self, and a satisfaction of both being accepted as a man and not being exposed as trans. For those who undertake a medical transition with a focus on shifting their bodies to more comfortable alignment with their inner gender awareness, body image and appearance are important early transition issues that can lead to increased life satisfaction.

Immediately at the end of his story Ed connected the shirt-off experience to that of his past and said: "I wish that all women could experience that feeling of just being able to take your shirt off and have it not be a big deal, you know. Yeah, it really shouldn't be, but it is." Here he spoke almost as an advocate when he wished all women could have a similar experience; from his new position as a man he reflected on the benefits that this freedom could have for women within a patriarchal regime that controls women's public attire. This reflects perhaps the sexist and cultural restrictions he resented previously in his female-bodied presentation that he was free of as a trans man. Still, that Ed thought of this as an option, however improbable, was an indicator that he had not forgotten his pre-transition experience when he performed in a female social gender role.

Like a number of the guys I spoke with, gender was something Ed was aware of for most of his life, although the idea of transgender was something that he did not understand until he was in his later twenties. Before this, transgender and transition were not options of which Ed had conceived, or had thought might address some tensions within him. As an abusive relationship with a non-trans woman came to an end – one that caused a six-year rift between Ed and his parents – Ed shared that what became available was the psychic space for him to finally consider transition; until then the relationship had taken up all of that space. His relatively short, two-year transition process included the testosterone-therapy-and-chest-surgery combination that all trans men in this study had chosen for themselves and had successfully accessed; like some others, Ed had also had a hysterectomy.

Having the support of his re-established parental relationship, the stability of a well-paid, unionized blue-collar job, and a comfortable and affordable condo, Ed reflected on his own satisfaction:

> I own my own home, um, which is relatively new. Having my
> mom and my dad in my life and having them be so positive and
> such a big part of my life now is so fantastic. It makes me

incredibly happy. You know, the friends that I have in my life
are people that I can have in my life until I die, until they die,
whoever goes first. I never really felt that before.

Home, family and friends are staples in anyone's life and key to
individuals' sense of stability in their lives. Here Ed spoke with
confidence about home ownership and implied the protection that it
affords him. He spoke of his parents and friends as playing a
significant role in his life today and in the future. And then he said he
had never felt this way before about his relationships.

In terms of the personal supports and resources that improved
Ed's transition experience, he explained that the stability afforded by
family and friends was one important factor in his satisfying life, and
there were others.

I have a good job. It's not the greatest job in the world but
excitement-wise it's kind of dull but it's an excellent job. It's
good pay, it's great benefits, it's, you know, it's secure, which
right now [in a Recession] I know everybody is freaking out
about their jobs and positions and lifestyle. So really, yeah, it's
all of those things, um, that are part of my life that make me
incredibly happy. Uh, you know, what makes me usually
satisfied, comfortable.

Ed's story speaks to the everyday desires that many of us have. Ed
spoke about some of his more conventional goals and desires in terms
of job, home and social relationships. This yearning for 'normalcy' is
consistent with conversations I have had with other post-transition

trans men and, to me, it comes across as a 'keeping-up-with-the-Joneses' desire to catch up with male peers in terms of career advancement, family evolvement, and social integration. Ed's blue-collar pragmatism shone through in his reflection that his employment represents personal security, particularly in light of current economic uncertainty. He acknowledged the working-class compromise he made in taking a great job that is also "dull," and seemed to accept this compromise.

What I would highlight here is how conventional are Ed's desires for family and community and stability. I believe that much of the social construction of the trans experience, at least the non-trans perspective of the trans experience, is that trans people's lives are significantly different from those of non-trans people. What Ed's story reveals, and a common thread through the stories shared by the men I talked with for this book, is that for the most part these trans lives are quite ordinary.

Ed continued to speak about his current sense of satisfaction: I like who I am. I like who I'm becoming. Um, and although I'm not, when I say 'becoming' actually I'm sort of pretty much there now. You know, physically I very, very slowly change still. And I don't know at what point changes stop, you know, after you do testosterone for how many years? You know, maybe I'll eventually get a little hairy chest. I have no idea [laughs]. Right now I've got, like, six or seven hairs [laughs].

Ed acknowledged that his transition was not a discrete process; while he was "pretty much there," small shifts were continuing to occur that may have had to do with ongoing and regular use of testosterone, and/or the relationship of this to aging. Here, also, Ed's 'trans-adolescence' emerged as he wished for more chest hair, a common masculine gender marker. His tone conveyed a lack of stress about this that was likely related to the previous story where he was convinced by the reactions of a carload of girls that his chest does, in fact, 'pass.'

What seemed to surprise Ed was what he heard and did not hear at the larger group meeting he attended:

> Listening to the other people talking about some of their past and where they had been and how people have related to them and where they are at present, I guess it may not necessarily be fair for me to say but I actually didn't really get a really great sense that some of the people were satisfied with their life at this point...Satisfaction with your life is all relative to how your life has been, right? And but I just sort of, I expected to feel more satisfaction coming from the individuals because from your original [recruitment] email, you were looking for people who were really satisfied with their lives the way they turned out and stuff. And it just, I just didn't get that from everyone.

Interesting here was Ed's need to quantify satisfaction; he thought that the men who would participate in a project like this would clearly be more satisfied than he observed. At the same time he revealed some of his criteria for gauging satisfaction when he said that it is "all relative." Apparently what he heard at the group meeting did not provide enough information for him to see how far the other guys had come in their own journeys; while they spoke of their milestones, there was seemingly not enough information about the length of their journey. This highlights for me the highly personal nature of 'subjective well-being' and our desire to compare ourselves to others and, in some cases, disbelieve and deny others their self-proclaimed contentment.

For Ed, his satisfaction was based on the ease with which he has been able to proceed through his transition and the final results. In discussing this with me, he seemed to develop some insights into why others' experiences of contentment may be different:

> I feel for myself that the way everything has come together for me, uh, has been hugely satisfying. I feel very lucky because I feel like it's been incredibly easy for me and I know it hasn't been that way for many people. Perhaps that's part of the lack of satisfaction I hear or that I'm picking up.

I am curious about how Ed attempted to come to terms with and understand his own "easy" course through transition as compared to the more challenging experiences of others. For Ed, how much did this ease contribute to his satisfaction, and did he perceive a more difficult transition as being less satisfying?

He was not so sure that the difficulties experienced by other trans people, or queer people for that matter, was all that different from that which non-trans and non-queer folks experience:

If you're talking about stress, I just... you know, people that think LGBT, all those letters together...[and that] we have a harder time, [and] maybe some of us do. But then there's some straight people out there, an awful lot of them that are having equally hard times and harder times. Personally I think really the stress that we as individuals feel regardless of what gender preferences we prefer or what gender we are or are becoming, I find for myself that it takes a lot to stress me out. I don't get stressed out about much. I don't get upset about much. In fact, if nothing else, I think that initially when I started taking testosterone, it calmed me down.

Interesting here is the connection Ed drew to the initiation of HRT. Like two other guys, he spoke of it as calming; another fellow said starting testosterone made him feel "more natural." There was no consensus on this particular topic as others spoke of testosterone's energizing, sexually-arousing and sometimes emotionally-agitating effects. I do believe that Ed's story raises questions about the effects of testosterone because it is contrary to general thought, questions that would benefit from greater research.

Ed seemed to vacillate between a belief that queer and trans people have a "harder time" and his perception that everyone can experience difficulties in their lives. He saw stress as an important factor, perhaps more important than gender and sexuality. I am reminded here about the impacts of stigma and wonder if Ed, like academics and others before him, was struggling to understand the impacts of the varying levels of stigma on people's lives.

More recently, Ed was looking for a primary relationship. Although he has been in relationships exclusively with non-trans women until now, he said he is now more focused on the individual, regardless of gender.

> I don't think it has anything to do with transitioning per se, but I think I've sort of gotten to a point where it doesn't really matter to me anymore if I meet somebody, whoever that somebody is, regardless of their gender. If I connect with that person then, then I'll see where it goes.

Ed seemed to be saying two things: first, that it does not matter if he starts another relationship and, second, that the gender of that person is less important than other factors. As our interview continued he clearly contradicted the first point: he does indeed want a relationship. What seemed to be more important was that Ed is coming to terms with how his experience of gender may interplay with the gender of a future partner. Ed is also understandably wary about engaging in a relationship due to bad relationship experiences in the past, but his life might be better, more satisfying, were he in relationship.

My other impression of Ed's statement, based on my experiences with gay men, was that this was a 'coming out' of sorts for Ed. The softened, vulnerable tone of his voice as he spoke of the possibility of being in relationship with a gay man reminded me of many conversations with friends and clients as they explored their own sexual identity. Here I believe it was my own identity as a gay man that contributed to, and allowed space and safety for, this sharing of information. "Who's the man?" Ed thought after a rousing chorus of flirts from a carload of girls. I wondered how Ed's constructions of 'man' and masculinity might be complicated by the possibility of accepting a gay or queer identity, and if his tentativeness was in part a reflection of that recognition.

> But there remained an issue he was working to overcome: I lack sexual confidence, you know. As long as I'm fully dressed, I feel great [laughs]. If I'm wearing my [underwear], I still feel fine but...it's just...knowing, removing that last piece and missing [a penis]. I guess, is important, you know [pause]. A lot of guys manage to work through it. I'm still working through that.

Where Ed would at another point in the interview express self-assurance in taking off his shirt after his encounter with the young women, here he expressed a lack of confidence at not having a penis, a primary marker of masculinity and of being a man.

Ed has clearly identified for himself an issue that is inhibiting his experience of intimacy. His experience was that other trans men have come to terms with this and he sees the need to grow in that direction. Implicit in this is also the need for trans men to manage information and disclosure of their trans-ness.

Other guys spoke of similar issues related to body image and sexual confidence and found themselves in different places along the continuum of comfort with themselves. For one fellow this was related to a self-described food addiction, another to disclosure of being trans to prospective sexual partners. Eric, who I will introduce later in this chapter, spoke clearly about a shift from being apologetic about his body toward a more matter-of-fact disclosure in the interest of not wanting to waste a potential lover's or his own time. Ed explained that some of the confidence he is lacking can be attributed to the previously described abusive relationship, an experience he clearly did not want to repeat.

Ed spoke of embracing and integrating the person he was prior to his transition:

> And I don't ever want to turn my back on who I was. I think that's a very, very important part of just being able to [pause] to survive happily. It's a huge part of my life that I'm satisfied with that. If I wasn't this person growing up, I wouldn't be this person that I am right now. I know there's guys out there that they don't acknowledge their history. And they don't seem to be happy either because they're always trying to hide something and it's just like there's nothing. Just be who you are and be comfortable with it. Accept what you've got. We do things [like HRT and surgery] to change, try and make ourselves a little bit more comfortable in our bodies. I look at that as being a slightly different thing.

Significant here, in my opinion, was Ed's perspective on medical procedures as they relate to the person he was. He spoke about his chest surgery, and later his hysterectomy and oophorectomy as a means of making the experience of his body more comfortable. For Ed, being more comfortable with his body seemed to be, in part, about revealing himself in different situations, like he did in a rural area outside of Vancouver, and experiencing the acceptance of his new identity. This story suggests the importance of integrating prior life and experience in order to improve well-being and, for friends, allies and other trans people, a red flag is raised for those trans men who might want to deny their prior experiences.

Ed's story demonstrated to me that some trans men do indeed have a positive transition experience that contributes to a satisfied life post-transition. The story he shared about being seen by the young women in the car demonstrated the importance of embodying the transition experience as a subjective, rather than medical, journey. He spoke of the significant support he received from family and friends, the meaning of having stability in housing and employment, and that, all in all, the issues he faced and values he expressed are rather commonplace. Ed charted for himself a rather conventional course and found himself a satisfying life.

In the next story, I will describe how another fellow came to recognize that there were two different stories about what transition was supposed to be like and how, through meeting a particular group of post-transition trans men, found the incentive to shift how he proceeded through his own transition.

KALEB'S STORY

The "Guys in the Woodwork"

Kaleb, a mid-thirties trans man, described himself as being eight years post-transition. He worked in a helping profession and stated at first contact how thrilled he was that a School of Social Work was conducting this kind of "positive research." Kaleb was the first but not the only person to describe a group of trans men who are no longer associated with trans communities and hold a particular kind of transition story. Until he met these men Kaleb felt frustrated with the negative stories he was hearing about transition equally from trans peers and service providers. After hearing positive stories Kaleb became hopeful for the first time, his transition experience made a significant shift and, as he explained, the process began working out much better for him.

> I finally found a couple of guys who actually came out of the woodwork to talk to me. And that was when I got to hear the positive stories, the hopeful stories. And once I got to hear their journeys, that was when I started to feel positive. And once I started to feel positive, then things started rolling.

Significant in this quote was that Kaleb said that he "started to feel positive" as this was indicative of a shift towards a better mental health. He went on to say that it was with this shift of feeling and state of mind that the activities of transition started falling into place. Again this points to the importance of maintaining a positive outlook on the transition experience and that the challenge of doing so is directly related to the dominant, negative narrative that trans men endure and that some trans men also perpetuate. Where were these "men in the woodwork" with their positive stories when Kaleb first began his transition? Clearly Kaleb did not hear their voices when he first began his journey, but eventually he overcame this obstacle.

Kaleb was able to name and describe most clearly what he called the "negative transition story," one to which almost everyone referred, a narrative that is portrayed in the support groups and by the medical establishments as the path every trans man should expect to be his own:

> When I came out and started, I was told [by peers], "No one is going to approve you. We've been trying for years so don't get your hopes up about getting any [testosterone] or surgery here..." The message that I got early on was just, "You're going to be unhappy. You're going to be stuck in a middle place because if they approve anything, it will only be half. So you'll be stuck in the middle, if you're lucky to even get that far, or you won't get anything."

This story was so vivid as Kaleb described it. The tone of his voice sounded disappointed and the sense I had was that he had hoped for more optimism, encouragement and support. Instead of hearing what the possibilities were, he heard about the limitations. What was missing for Kaleb, something that he did not know but seemed to sense, was that there was another perspective on how to proceed through transition in a much more positive way. Perhaps the conflict was with his state of mind: Kaleb seemed to be the kind of person who sets goals and follows through, so he was responding to the information, as well as the perspective of the individuals who were sharing it; he had just as much difficulty accepting the facts as he did their worldview. Had they spoken of challenges, possible solutions and exceptions to these outcomes he might have responded differently.

Kaleb clarified that the so-called 'middle place' he mentioned above was one where a trans person might be approved for hormones, but end up on a seemingly eternal waiting list for surgeries. But this was just the medical component; there were further repercussions based on the input from other trans people:

> [They said:] "No one is going to want to date you at all, especially if you're into men. Gay men will not want to date you so don't ever expect on dating or sleeping with a gay man" – which is bullshit. Sorry, excuse my language but it's absolute bullshit that gay men don't date and sleep with trans guys. But this is what I was told. So I had this vision of my life as being alone, miserable, depressed in a physical state that I didn't want to be in and just very unhappy. And, and I was going to be ridiculed.

After being told that he would not be able to access the health care that he desired, Kaleb was informed that he would also be socially isolated. Kaleb was angry. There was a shift in his tone and his use of the word 'bullshit' revealed his growing frustration at the time as well as his hindsight perspective. As he recalled his experiences, his affect suggested that he was counseling an earlier version of him, sending a message to himself at that time that there were other options, and that the messages he received really were "bullshit."

As though the medical and social ramification were not enough for Kaleb to contend with, he was also forewarned about the perceptions of employers in terms of mental health and substance abuse.

> Oh, "You're going to lose your job." I heard from medical professionals and the community that, "No trans guy can successfully transition at work." Yeah and, "All trans guys have mental health and [alcohol and drug problems]." [pause] I heard all these things and I'm finding that none of them are applicable to my life now.

Kaleb described more of these allegedly definitive outcomes, the unavoidable experiences that every trans man must endure. He expressed his frustration at hearing no alternatives to unsuccessful transition. From a place of hindsight, he stated that these issues were not, and have not been, for him, significant during or post-transition. For Kaleb, this list of outcomes that the "negative transition story" predicted instead became a survey of experiences that he avoided and, in part, I expect some of his motivation through transition came from a desire to prove that story wrong. He would proceed through transition differently.

So who were these people from whom Kaleb eventually heard a different transition narrative? Kaleb introduced the idea of the 'guys in the woodwork.' I asked him to clarify who they were and their significance:

> After about six or eight months I got wind that, that there were the 'guys in the woodwork.' That's what I ended up calling them – 'the guys in the woodwork' – because they certainly weren't at any trans event or social or support group. So, I made it my mission to find them 'cause I thought, "these guys are my answer." I actually found these 'guys in the woodwork.' And these were guys who transitioned five, ten, fifteen, twenty years ago and are very happy and content in their lives and got through their transitions despite what the professionals will sometimes tell you, or guys in the community will sometimes tell you. It is possible to move through the process in a good timely manner with lots of support.

At this point in the interview Kaleb clarified that for the first six or eight months after his decision to transition he actually believed the "negative transition story." There was optimism in his tone when he spoke about discovering that there was another story and it became the focus of his transition from that point forward. What I learned was that, contrary to the dominant assumption that transition must be situated within a medical and health context, Kaleb stated clearly that a phase of his transition consisted of seeking out trans men with positive stories so that he could make different choices about how he would engage in his own transition.

Kaleb spent the first six to eight months of his transition searching for answers because it was clear to him that stories he was hearing were not quite right. The messages he was getting from the community were not consistent with his worldview and it was only when he met the 'men in the woodwork' that he finally heard some positive stories. His experience put the subjective experience of the transition journey in the foreground. This differs from health literature and popular discourse about transition that focuses on medical and psychiatric aspects of transition. In terms of mental health, a positive outlook can have a significant effect on the experience and success that trans men will have. Kaleb was not the only one to highlight the merits of a positive outlook on life in relation to a successful transition. This suggests that not only can the "negative transition story" be a barrier, but also that an optimistic approach to transition can improve the mental health outcomes and sense of satisfaction for trans men.

Kaleb stated that once he sensed an internal shift from a negative to a positive attitude that was when he recognized he was in control of his transition and became assertive about starting the medical components of it. "I got on testosterone, I got my surgeries – with a lot of guilt mind you... [laughter] 'cause guys that lived here five, you know eight years before me were still on waitlists for surgeries." Kaleb's reference to guilt combined with the laughter that followed expressed the degree of his discomfort in knowing that he had managed to get his needs met while others were still struggling to do the same. Kaleb understood that he had socio-economic advantages that made accessing surgeries easier for him, and he was only one of many to describe the guilt that interfered with these post-transition trans men's present-day participation in trans communities. They speak of the negative stories they hear at the groups and yet by not returning with positive stories they perpetuate exactly what they found problematic. They spoke of their desire to be involved, and then an inability to do so. Later, I will report on another fellow, Eric, who described more broadly the experience of guilt and its ramifications. I believe the reason many of these trans men no longer associated with trans men communities was in part due to a perspective that they had completed their transitions and that they were no longer seen as trans. Perhaps they saw trans communities as people sharing the sole interest of transition and simply found little use for these groups anymore. Or perhaps they preferred to move away from situations that reminded them of the ease with which they transitioned, while others continued to struggle.

Based on information Kaleb gleaned from these 'guys in the woodwork', he recognized that there was a game that he needed to play in order to get the health care he wanted:

> At the gender clinic...they expected me to be depressed. And
> I went in there not depressed [laughter]. But I kind of got the
> message from some of 'the guys in the woodwork' [that] you

have to play the suicide game. And I wasn't suicidal but I had to pretend I was a five [out of ten] on the suicide scale. [I thought], "Oh I'm going to have to hone my inner acting abilities from high school" because if you weren't, then they weren't going to approve you for anything... I had to play the suicide game and I thought, "This is ridiculous. This is so bad that I have to pretend that I'm this suicidal to get you to say yes to something." I had all the guys tell me, "Oh, your doctor is not going to say yes."...It's crazy how many people expect you to be that depressed and suicidal whether it's the peer support from the community, whether it's psychiatrists from the old gender clinic. It's crazy how depressed you have to be to prove that you're trans, that you're really a four or five on our trans bullshit scale.

This powerful narrative reveals how Kaleb and the Woodworkers colluded to undermine the systemic barriers they faced and take control of their healthcare through an act of resistance. In a way they had developed a variation on the script by which the healthcare providers were expecting them to play. Without a doubt, any mention of a "suicide game" can be dangerous. Kaleb and the others would not be expected to understand the responsibilities a social worker would have to support the positive mental health and well being of their clients, particularly those who may be exhibiting signs of suicide. They have no need to consider the legal and ethical responsibilities and balance these with the right to self-determination of clients while considering clients' capacity to make decisions for themselves. To introduce an additional factor, a game where clients are 'acting out' suicidal ideation is unnecessary; clients should be able to speak openly about their mental health. Kaleb was not the only one to describe how he influenced his health care. Another spoke of web sites accessible only to trans men which list service providers and wherein trans community members recommend language, behavior, style of dress and affect that they believed that these providers were seeking and what they thought might lead these providers to deny trans men the services that they sought. These are the kinds of obstacles that the men felt that they had to conquer.

Kaleb's story revealed the magnitude of the "negative transition story" and the multiple realms on which it can have an impact: social supports, relationships, housing and employment are all potentially at jeopardy, but this is not a foregone conclusion. It was in response to the many manifestations of the "negative transition story" that he demonstrated the resilience and coping strategies he needed to persevere with his decision. In the next story I illustrate some of the impacts that the "negative transition story" can have on one individual's mental health and wellness. As we will see, in Eric's case it presented a significant barrier and added complexity to maintaining his mental health as well as his sobriety.

ERIC'S STORY

The bright orange egg

In his first contact with me Eric first stated clearly that he would not have taken part, or even opened the email describing the project, had it not been for the direct suggestion of another trans man who vouched for me as an ally. Like all of the men I spoke with, he described a rather quick progression of less than two years from his decision to transition to completing the process. For him, this involved TRT, chest contouring, hysterectomy and oophorectomy.

A former substance abuser with four years of sobriety prior to starting transition, Eric reported that every day for the first year of his gender transition he carried a small orange plastic egg (such as those found in *Kinder Surprise* chocolate treats). Inside, rather than a toy or puzzle, it contained a mix of illicit drugs. One might immediately think this was a foolish idea on his part; indeed, even Eric questioned the merits of that decision. He quite deliberately and thoughtfully described how he came to carry the drugs with him:

> It was hard in the beginning not to, [pause] not to go back to using drugs... At one point early in my transition I was so close to using drugs again. I started actually carrying them around with me. I'm not sure what part of my brain thought that was a good idea, but I sort of had this idea that one day very soon I was definitely going to need to do it. And I didn't want to have to, like, freak out 'cause I didn't have any access [laughs] to drugs.

In retrospect, Eric questioned the cognitive process that brought him to purchasing crystal methamphetamine, ecstasy and some unidentified prescription medications, and carrying these around with him in a bright orange egg. He told me that every evening he would empty his pockets, including the egg, and every morning tuck the egg back in. Particularly in the beginning weeks and months of his transition, he felt that returning to substance abuse was not just a possibility, but a certainty. He described his relationship to substance use in terms of spatial and temporal proximity; he was "so close", and at times he spoke of the immediacy in terms of hours. Despite a four-year abstinence, as he began transition he said the balance his life, career and relationships family members still felt "precarious"; to transition might risk upsetting this tenuous balance further. Substances had been a way he had coped with these in the past.

Eric never did open the egg. "One day I [thought], 'this is a really fuckin' bad idea' [*laughs*]. And that was that! I got rid of them and that was that." Eric had been so certain he was "definitely going to need" the drugs to help manage anxiety, so what happened? There was no grand drama, as he had expected. He had managed to prevail over the difficulties he had faced early in his transition. The drugs had been available to help him cope with the transition-related challenges that he had been convinced would arise. A year later, when these challenges had not materialized and he was feeling more satisfied with his life, he simply disposed of the egg. "I didn't think I was ever going to tell [that story to] anybody. It's interesting."

Eric's successful negotiation of the health care system did not come without its challenges, as he explained:

Everything happened very quickly and I felt guilty about that. And I sort of still do because I didn't spend a lot of time really talking with other trans people about their transitions. I did a fair amount of listening, and then...all of these people, so many people couldn't get testosterone or couldn't actually take it for some medical or whatever reason. It's sort of the medical path; usually the first step is testosterone. And so many people were having trouble with [accessing testosterone], not to mention the hysterectomy, the chest surgeries and the lower surgeries, and how long people were waiting. And I think that, to be honest, it's like a big part of why I disengaged from everything. And, I know lots of people who are four, five, six, seven years or more who still haven't had surgery. So I guess... [pause] There's guilt that I deal with that I think I'm always going to. And I think [that guilt is] always going to prevent me from sharing to some degree. I mean it might just, um, my story is sort of, I tell it differently depending on who's listening. [looks at recording device] Um, but I'm trying really hard not to think about who's listening right now [laughs]. It's just you.

The guilt Eric described, much like Kaleb, is in response to the "negative transition story," within which he saw others trapped while he was able to progress. In Eric's case, he paid for some of the surgeries out of his own pocket. He had the resources to ensure his transition would be successful. Eric's discomfort seemed in part to be situated in the awareness of his own economic and class-based privilege. One could argue that even with the challenges of transphobia, he experienced easier access to healthcare services because he was white, college-educated, possessed strong English language skills and had the financial resources to pay for service. The same could be said for most of the trans men in this project, although having class-based privilege does not necessarily removed systemic barriers as much as it reduces them.

Eric was aware of his social location within the discourse about transition, and the "negative transition story" in particular. He saw himself in relation to that story and at the same time separated from trans men's communities by the fact that his own story did not match the negative narrative. The institutional structure of the health care system, by limiting access to transition-related services, perpetuated the isolation and contributed to the misery of those other trans men, those still waiting "four, five, six, seven years or more" for services. Eric saw me as a researcher and ally in another, separate role; while speaking to a queer man, he was more at ease and less inhibited by guilt and made efforts to not censor his story despite his aware of the recording device on the desk between us.

Eric acknowledged that his success came in part due to his

sobriety at the time he began his transition. Four years prior he had stopped using a mix of prescription and recreational drugs when he realized the negative impact they were having on his life. He quit 'cold turkey.' On reflection he stated:

> The idea of transitioning in the middle of all that...[*pause*] would not have been helpful. I likely would have not ended up clean or transitioning [*laughs*]. It would have been some sort of nasty death spiral [*laughs*]. Um, fortunately I deal...I dealt with my substance issues a lot, like several years before I started transitioning.

Interesting here was the slip in language (one I would have missed were it not for my astute transcriber). He clearly spoke in the present tense when he said, "fortunately I deal", and then shifted into the past tense and restated the word as "dealt." While perhaps not in the forefront of his current life, I interpreted this to mean that he maintained some conscious awareness that his substance abuse was to some degree an ongoing issue. In terms of the realms of his life that Eric reviewed in assessing his subjective well-being, clearly his sobriety was among them. Furthermore, in retrospect, Eric was aware of the ramifications had he misused substances while in transition: probably neither sobriety nor transition would have been successfully achieved.

Like many might, I believed in the inadvisability of carrying the egg until my advisor asked if there was another way I might understand it. Indeed, had the egg been empty, I could imagine it as a talisman that offered comfort to someone who felt quite alone on his journey toward finding himself. He navigated his own path and took along with him a talisman for protection and, while he appreciated the security of having it, he neither opened it, nor consumed its contents. So what difference would it make what was inside? By carrying around this egg, Eric put himself at risk for legal troubles and relapse, but at the end of that journey he was just fine. Eric made choices, some wise, others perhaps inadvisable, but whatever the combination, he eventually reached a place of contentment some years ago.

Eric, like Kaleb and some of the other guys, credited some of his success to having heard positive transition stories from post-transition trans men. These 'stories from the woodwork' were the exception, and not easy to come by as the individuals sharing them were difficult to locate. After finally hearing these stories, Eric and a close friend decided they would stop attending a popular peer support group in order to dislodge themselves from the downbeat stories, and to make their own path.

Eric's story demonstrated not just his ability to cope with the pressure of the "negative transition story," pressure that was magnified by a history of problematic substance use, but also how misinforming that story can be. How much did that pressure impact his decision to pay for his own surgeries and bypass the system of transition, and many of his peers within it, just to avoid the added burden of that route? What might be different if perspectives on the medical transition shifted and were more in line with Eric's personal intention; would it be possible to conceive of HRT and surgeries as enjoyable, positive experiences for those who choose them. While I expect most trans men might be contented to undergo medical procedures because they are eager for the results, can enjoyment be found in the journey as well as the destination?

Weaving the stories together

The themes I present are broad, reaching across this group of trans men, while the stories I have shared are as unique as the individuals they represent and speak to a subgroup of trans men who have made particular choices around how they would proceed with their transitions, choices many others make differently. These stories are neither intended to demonstrate how all trans men undertake transition, nor provide evidence for how trans men *should* do this. Instead, I have used selected stories from my conversations with trans men to illuminate some of the key ideas I took from my experiences with them. I elaborate on these further in the next chapter.

There are two competing narratives about transition that the trans men in this project shared about their mental health and wellness. In the first, as Ed and the others demonstrated, much like the 'men in the woodwork'" before them, many trans men have satisfying, perhaps even conventional lives. They found satisfaction after prevailing over the challenges of early transition and despite the louder rival narrative in the "negative transition story" that Kaleb and others so effectively described, wherein trans men are pathologized unwitting victims at the mercy of healthcare professionals and society, destined to live miserable lives. The potential impacts of this latter narrative are immense, and speak to the strength and self-efficacy of those who do successfully maneuver through their individual transition process, however they charted their own course. In this book we read about bold, transgressive acts that undermined the systemic barriers they faced and subverted the dominant medical narrative. Supports and resources made constructive contributions to these men's lives, and although partners and families were key for some, for others it was the kindness of strangers that made a difference. Having access to class-based resources such as money, education and language made a key difference for some. Ultimately it seems vital that trans men who complete their transitions share their stories in order to give hope to other trans men, however many guys and the 'men in the woodwork' are reluctant to do so.

The men I spoke with assessed their life satisfaction in many common ways. They valued maintaining social relationships and having stable employment and housing. More challenging for some individuals were the negative social forces, particularly those implicated in the "negative transition story," and how these exacerbated anxiety for those who did not have strong coping strategies. For those with a history of problematic substance use, maintaining sobriety was a significant consideration. While some noted that their transition experiences had contributed to improved mental health and wellness, they were reluctant to speak about their experiences with others who were still transitioning despite knowing the benefits of sharing positive stories. In the next chapter I discuss possible reasons for their reluctance. I also consider the ramifications of these findings more broadly within the context of the present literature, both scientific and theoretical, and discuss how these could inform health and mental health practice.

5 | HOW THESE STORIES CHANGE OUR PRACTICE

Funny, heart-warming, difficult and curious were the stories I heard in March and April 2009 when I met eight generally-satisfied trans men from Vancouver and asked them to describe their journeys. We gathered in small groups at the offices of a local non-profit, and then I visited with each one-on-one, usually in their own homes. I heard about what made their lives so contented in the present, and their reflections on the challenges they had faced and managed. The findings demonstrate the complexity and contradictions experienced in these lives, and are not simply black and white narratives. With these stories in mind, I discuss here my interpretation of the issues.

I started this process by asking: what can be learned from the stories of trans men about their mental health and wellness? In relation to this, I was curious in which realms of trans men's lives is satisfaction important and/or significant? I answer these questions within three thematic areas. First I underscore the reality of their contentment with their own lives, and the realms of life they considered in their self-assessment of life satisfaction. Next I describe the impacts of the "negative transition story" on their lives. Finally, I explore how the tension between these two narratives resulted in these trans men becoming so alienated from their communities. Then I move on to discuss the significance of the my findings within the context of the present literature on subjective well-being and quality of life, and theories of identity development. I discuss implications for strengths-based social work practice and introduce an assessment tool that I created for health providers and addictions counsellors to explore with trans men some of their transition-related issues.

What We Learn About the Lives of Trans Men
The road to satisfaction

The guys described a number of factors that contributed to their life satisfaction, some rather commonplace, others more unique. Like many, having access to healthcare, resources and social supports made a difference in being able to ease through transition. For those with a history of problematic substance use, ongoing sobriety was key. As trans men, the desire for friendship with other trans men, and partnership was important. They recognized the benefit of overcoming intimacy and body-image issues and reaching greater comfort with their own bodies. Integration of pre- and post-transition selves was a significant issue for these trans men.

These men demonstrated that it is indeed possible to be a

contented and happy trans man, although each individual described this experience uniquely. In three cases they set as an intent quite early on that they would undertake their transitions differently, perhaps enjoyably. In four cases, they spent the first six to eight months seeking out a different way to go about transition because their experiences did not match the negative stories of others. Most eventually found 'men in the woodwork' from whom they finally heard some positive stories. They wanted to hear from others who had found their way through the healthcare system. They sought stories that might help them find the intrinsic motivation and ways to proceed with transition on their own terms. These stories highlighted the personal part of the transition journey, a divergence from the healthcare literature and the popular discourse about transition that focuses on the medical and the psychiatric experience.

These men each demonstrated a degree of personal dedication in deciding to go about their transitions in their own way. They each shifted their transition into a personally controlled experience rather than relying on a medically-prescribed performance of transition. They challenged the implicit bias in stories that suggest 'completing' transition as an idealized experience that necessitates all trans men undergo HRT and have both top and bottom surgeries. This bias demeans those who do not choose that path, making them lesser trans persons, and encumbers them with expectations regarding the hormonal and surgical steps they should take; further it ignores that some trans men may feel quite content solely with HRT and, being comfortable with their bodies as they are, have no need for surgery. Legal status and documents notwithstanding, newly transitioning trans men need to know that any point on the transition spectrum can be an end-point and is perfectly valid and legitimate. Further, they can choose to shift along the spectrum at their own pace if they have the resources to afford the time and surgery costs. Ultimately these men were able to take control of their own lives and decision-making, and demonstrate self-efficacy in their negotiations of the medical system.

The "negative transition story"

The "negative transition story" is a socially constructed and highly problematic narrative that insists that being trans means having had life-long gender identity disorder, and mental health and addiction issues. Individuals will lose their social supports, housing, and employment, and find accessing healthcare, including transition, daunting if not impossible. This story, perpetuated by trans and non-trans people, peers and providers alike, is so convincing that some resorted to extreme measures in order to manage their anxiety when pre-existing coping strategies were limited. The potential impacts on mental health and wellness in trans men's communities include significantly increased anxiety and stress.

The challenges they faced when accessing health care, while real and substantial, were a symptom of a greater systemic problem, and they recognized they could change that story. Rather than accepting this narrative as the only outcome for their experience, they resisted and chose a different path. They demonstrated a greater sense of contentment when asked about life satisfaction, and were able to consider medical gender transition among a larger list of options.

At its core the message of the "negative transition story" seems to be that transition will lead to misery; further, the primary purpose of the "negative transition story" is to maintain the problematic gender binary: There are only two 'natural' genders – natal men and women – and life satisfaction can only be experienced from either of these two biocentric poles. Any degree of variance from these positions brings with it an associated and appropriate level of stigma, discontent and misery. Further, even those trans men whose transitions achieve convincing masculine appearances could never be content because they have undermined the essential sex to which they were assigned at birth. This story highlights the investment that some members of trans communities have in maintaining this narrative, and their perception of health-care providers' similar participation.

Two narratives converge

A peculiar dichotomy exists in the experience of post-transition trans men and their relationships to trans communities. Participants spoke of the significance of hearing positive transitions stories and yet found these stories hard to come by. They spoke about frustration and guilt when considering their own experiences compared to other trans men they knew. Participants met the 'guys in the woodwork' and then became them. Like those men, participants had distanced themselves from trans communities. They expressed guilt with their own perceived ease at completing transition and their moving on to a satisfied life while others have been unable to do so.

I believe that this guilt stemmed from an awareness, overt or not, of the numerous social disparities that prevent equal access to and experience of gender transition. For example, being of a lower class and living in a less affluent socio-economic situation could prevent access to trans-related health care simply for financial reasons, even if partially subsidized by medical insurance. When I asked what participants could do to help disseminate positive stories, they said they were willing to tell their stories, but only if asked.

'Transgender readability privilege' (TRP) is the language I use to describe the confluence of factors like race, class, biological and genetic predispositions that make social interactions easier for some than others within a Western society because others perceive them more easily as the affirmed gender. Here I use the word 'read' as an interpretation that may or not be the intent of the individual in question. There are many influencing factors and I highlight only a few here. For example, being white, being of a particular class that a person can afford to transition, and/or also having the physiology and genetic makeup that allows for HRT to work effectively so that facial hair and other more obvious markers of masculinity help individuals to be recognized as men. Race and ethnicity create additional barriers to healthcare for men of colour, particularly those of Black, Asian and First Nations ethnicity described herein, and in terms of how the markers of masculinity are racialized as white and set differently for these trans men. Class-based implications include the affordability of HRT and surgical costs as well as the time and ability to focus transition over other areas of life. The 'right' genetics and physiology combine with HRT can create a more convincing appearance of masculinity. TRP means people masculinize more quickly, and more effectively, because they have greater capacity to maneuver through the health care system and overcome trans-related barriers.

The positive experiences these trans men had during transition collided with the "negative transition story" and contributed to them moving away from trans communities. As they observed others caught up in that narrative, just as they themselves had been at one time, they could not figure out how to talk about a different way through transition. Participants knew how helpful hearing positive stories were in their own experience, yet could not find ways to pass them on. Guilt and privilege seem implicated here, and yet these are issues that a community should be able to manage with extant resources. Their participation in a research study like this one demonstrates willingness and a desire to change the dominant story, however strategies are needed that these trans men can employ.

I highlight this issue of guilt not to admonish these trans men, but rather to underscore the disparity between these men and the vast majority of others. These participants were a rarity in that, for the most part, they had all undergone 'top surgery' and some form of 'bottom' surgery and had a high degree of socio-economic privilege;

they succeeded because they could afford the investment of time, energy and resources to get it done. I do not to deny them their accomplishments as they still had to overcome the systemic and social barriers all trans men face when they transition; this demonstrates their self-efficacy. Most trans men do not have the resources or social capital to reach this stage of transition, if they desire it.

In order to effect change in the lives of trans men, policy must make it easier to navigate the institutionalized gender transition systems. On a community level this means ensuring support programs and groups such as those described by participants are facilitated in such a way as to counter the "negative transition story." This does not mean that only positive accounts should be shared, but rather that challenges described by individuals are met with recommendations of strategies to overcome these, and culturally-competent professional intervention when necessary. Indeed, by investing more resources into transgender healthcare and mental health care that make access easier, we can reduce the harmful impacts of systemic traumatization that may result in extended engagement in a medicalized transition model.

FINDINGS IN RELATION TO THE LITERATURE
A feminist lens on the lives of trans men

Scott-Dixon described the importance of framing 'trans' as "a social and political, rather than a medical and psycho-therapeutic, category" (p. 18), a lens which proved useful during this project. This shift in perspective brought to the forefront the stories these participants shared about the social experience of transition. In many cases their relationships with their families, friends and communities were difficult and challenging, but if the analysis stops there we are caught again in a circuit of pathology. As I describe in the next section, it was in part because of these experiences that participants showed how capable they were at setting goals for their transitions, and following through in the face of social and systemic adversity.

Raymond's (1994) perspective on 'transgender' demonstrates shortsightedness by focusing superficially on the components of transition: the clothing, hormones and surgical interventions. The men in this project spoke about these as issues that are part of a greater narrative of being seen socially as men and/or gender non-conforming people and the implications on their safety. Raymond would have been wise to look at how these implements of transition contribute to the experience of gender, and to consider Lorber's (2005) ideas in order to explore how the gender binary informs the medical and non-medical choices trans men make about transition. Lorber was correct in her assertion that the gender binary plays a role in transition in that it defines the categories with which these trans men negotiated in their search for contentment. As the scope of inquiry grows wider, the landscape of gender broadens and allows theorists unique opportunities to unpack the socially constructed roles we all play and the effects on trans men of having been socialized as girls and women, whether or not they experienced themselves in that way; as participants described, for some there was early awareness of discordant gender while for others there was not.

Findings from this project, particularly regarding the "negative transition story", support the research of Cole, Denny, Eyler and Samons (2000) and their assertions regarding the implications of language like 'disorder' and the ongoing pathologization of the medical model. Participants demonstrated the necessity of acknowledging what these authors referred to as "the in-between state" as a vital stop on their journeys, whether enjoyable or stressful. Like their early gendered socialization, these experiences needed to be integrated by participants in order to reach satisfied lives.

Satisfaction and subjective well-being

The overarching story shared by the trans men in this book is first and foremost that trans men can be satisfied with their lives and this is, according to my Advisory Group and participants, likely to be groundbreaking information for those invested in the dominant transition narrative. That this might be such a significant shift in thinking is something I can only attribute to the deep-seated societal belief in the pathology of trans people that stems from the historical institutionalization of 'trans as mental illness' in the *DSM*. Even as GID is replace in the manual with GD, I believe the lingering effects of 'trans as a diagnosis' will continue, much as we have seen with homosexuality's inclusion and ultimate removal from the *DSM* (for a comprehensive discussion of this issue, see Drescher, 2009). Heterosexism is a fundamental social structure that benefits certain groups, and is reproduced in education, religion, law, the arts, and health and social services. Similar structures continue to function in relation to gender and the clear lines between the sexes; patriarchy and heterosexism are two examples, and transphobia a third. The "negative transition story" is evidence that the medical institution considers trans men so mentally ill that the concept that they could be satisfied is a revelation. These men are satisfied not just because they responded to a recruitment ad that used satisfaction as a criteria; they demonstrated their satisfaction in ways that are rather commonplace and not particularly unique to trans people.

Diener's (1984) describes subjective well-being as having three criteria: it is assessed individually, comprises both helpful and lack of unhelpful factors, and is comprehensive. Participants provided critical self-assessments that were subjective, clearly situated in their lived experience, considered both negative and positive factors, and were global in nature. The road to satisfaction was not always well paved for these trans men but with the support of their social networks, positive stories from select peers, and demonstrated self-efficacy, they made their own way. They spoke about self-actualization, the importance of supportive relationships, and of having a sense of personal power. They had purpose in their lives and their reflections made it clear that they were invested in their personal growth.

Based on the realms of life described by Ryff (1989) – positive relations with others, self-acceptance, autonomy, environmental mastery, purpose in life, and personal growth – these men demonstrated self-acceptance in the decision to begin transition and in their present post-transition experience. They spoke of the value and the importance of their relationships with family members, parents, siblings, partners and close friends, and with work colleagues who do not know that they are trans. Each established autonomy by going his own way, defining his own path and working through medical transition in a way that was self-affirming. They reflected on the value of integrating their lives prior to transition and the meaning this had to them in the present. They stated a desire to positively influence the transition experience of others who might be struggling, even if only by changing the dominant narrative about it; their participation in this project is a demonstration of this intent. Moreover, many stated that participation in this project was a way for them to contribute meaningfully to trans communities and enabled them to reflect on their lives with others sharing similar experiences.

Thus, based on the criteria set out by Diener (1984) and Ryff (1989), these trans men are satisfied. They maintain relationships with family, friends and partners, have stable home and work environments and do well at managing the minor everyday stresses we all experience. The roads that these trans men have traveled to satisfaction have in many ways been different; here difference speaks to a trans experience as much as to the individuality we all possess, trans and non-trans alike. How their experiences are different due to gender transition can teach us a lot about how trans is socially constructed within our communities in general, and health care in particular.

Mental health and the *DSM*

Rarely does the health literature state that it is possible for trans men to move through transition in a good and timely manner with lots of support (Lev, 2004). For the men I spoke with, hearing positive stories from other trans men was incredibly helpful and thus the documenting of these positive transition stories is vital in order to dismantle the "negative transition story." These stories are in direct conflict with the dominant mental health framework, a hegemonic discourse that fosters a particularly unflattering narrative of transition with which trans men and service providers are forced to cope and contend. Documenting these stories is a first step toward shifting away from this troublesome narrative.

The *DSM-IV-TR* states "conflicts that are primarily between the individual and society are *not* mental disorders" (emphasis mine, American Psychiatric Association, 2000). Based on the stories shared here, the challenges and satisfaction trans men experience in their lives are predominantly a result of their social interactions, findings that support the work of Hansbury (2005) and Lawrence (2007).

With the release of the *DSM-V* expected in May, 2013, the diagnosis changes from Gender Identity Disorder (GID) to Gender Dysphoria (GD). The precise language will not be available until the actual release but the definition of GD is expected to reflect the emotional and psychological distress that results from a dissonance between one's affirmed gender (how I feel inside, whether or not I present as that gender) and the sex assigned at birth (the decision the doctor made based on what was between my legs). While the intent of this revision seems to be to allow for treatment without the stigma of a mental disorder, the ramifications remain to be seen. We do not yet know how mental health professionals who use the *DSM* will utilize the new guidelines, how quickly policies will be reviewed and revised, or how insurance companies will adjust their funding of services and procedures and impact access to healthcare for trans people. Even with the new term, GD, being trans remains a condition listed in the *DSM* and thus mental illness may still be inferred by those with a less sophisticated understanding of the purposes of the text, and potentially by politicians, lawyers and disgruntled spouses with ulterior motives. Other unanticipated outcomes, positive or negative, can't be ruled out.

The other challenges experienced by the trans men I have interviewed fall within the range of what a non-trans person might experience and are, for the most part, not related to transition or being trans, but rather to how society responds to their gender. For service providers this understanding is key to shifting trans-related mental health care away from *disorder*, and toward addressing the external factors that influence and impact the individual, cause depression, anxiety and other social stressors. By utilizing strengths-based practice (Saleebey, 1996) and understanding how trans men describe their subjective well-being, we can make significant inroads into improving access to mental health care. I provide an Assessment Tool in Chapter Six to assist in the evaluation of this impact.

Implications for Developmental and Identity Theory

Developmental and identity models by Lev (2004), Devor (2004) and Hansbury (2005) are helpful in unpacking some of the mental health issues presented by participants. Devor's (2004) discussion about the importance of mirroring provides insight into the frustration many participants shared about participating in trans communities and attending support groups. There they saw other attendees as witnesses, but did not desire them as mirrors; they preferred to model the "guys in the woodwork" as more successful, transitionally speaking. Located somewhere near Devor's tenth stage, *Delay before Transition,* and Lev's (2004) second phase of seeking information and reaching out, these men listened at the door of the trans community and heard the cacophony of the "negative transition story" and still persevered and moved ahead.

For some participants there seemed to be a further disjuncture between the stages of *Integration* and *Pride*: where does a trans man who is living stealth fit? How prideful is a trans man who is reluctant to share proactively his successful transition story with others? Separating from trans communities, or living stealth like the "guys the woodwork" is an option that some trans men choose. For the men who were the most disengaged from trans communities (despite participating in this project), there was clearly a sense of great satisfaction with life. Consistent with Hansbury's categories of identity (2005), these participants are more like the 'woodworkers' than 'transmen' or 'genderqueers' in that they identify as 'men,' live apart from the trans community and live rather conventional lives. Again, one must be cautious about any categorical assessment for the risk of created further binary thinking.

There is need to be cautious about using developmental models to create discrete and expected outcomes, and to recognize that trans men will move at different speeds and different ways along the spectrum. Language like 'success' and 'complete' in reference to transition need to be used cautiously, especially when they imply 'passing'. Some trans men may choose to not pass for personal or political reasons while others simply are not able to pass due to genetic factors and biological responses to HRT; for these individuals the stigma continues. Further, assessing completion in terms of gender performance is problematic, as Hansbury (2005) explains:

> The quandary is this: by setting up a system in which the final, triumphant goal is public pride and activism, FTMs who remain at the Integration stage – in the woodwork – may too easily be seen as developmentally stuck, as poor, misguided victims of the heteropatriarchy, suffering from internalized transphobia. (p.247)

'Woodworkers' I spoke with were neither developmentally stuck nor victims of heteropatriarchy thus sustaining Hansbury's caution. Some may be rightly concerned about how a person's mental health and well-being are affected when a large portion of their personal history and major milestones of their lives go unacknowledged, perhaps eventually becoming toxic. While I think 'hiding' may be harmful and that pride and activism can be beneficial, there is a space between these positions where a trans person may or may not disclose or act on political teaching moments presented in their everyday world.

Trans men in our project identified a wide range of life factors that related to their mental health and wellness. While identity models focus on the ramifications of being trans, they do not address all of a person's life. Transition-related concerns included: medical (hormones and surgeries) and non-medical transition options; 'passing'; trans-related 'coming out' to partners, friends and family, and concerns about loss of support; societal oppression due to transphobia; threats to socioeconomic security (e.g., housing, employment) because of discrimination; isolation and alienation; and internalized oppression. Issues identified by participants that were not specifically related to transition included: body image; concerns with aging; substance use and recovery; dating and relationships with non-trans people (heterosexual and lesbian women, gay and queer men); sexual intimacy issues; and concerns about long-term use of hormones. Models of trans-identity formation need to operate more holistically in order to incorporate this broader array of issues.

The concept of transition readability privilege (TRP) I described previously complements Krista Scott-Dixon's (2006) concept of 'gender privilege' in that it helps us understand why some trans men decide to disengage from trans communities. When trans men are read easily as men within society they have the option of not retaining their trans identity, at least socially. Some seem to assimilate and live plainly as men, while others maintain a trans identity. Thus trans men who pass benefit from gender-based privilege in contexts like the grocery store and classroom, but not in the bedroom and the doctor's office. Those who struggle to pass, or who only pass some of the time, find themselves less able to go about their lives, let alone access health services, without the burden of transphobia to influence interactions. Privilege is never all-encompassing and the subjective experience of privilege is always individual.

IMPLICATIONS FOR CLINICAL PRACTICE

When considering implications for health providers, I have different recommendations for generalist practice – the knowledge I would expect any health providers to have about trans people – than for specialist practitioners.

Strengths-based generalist practice with trans men

My hope is that providers need not just a general awareness of transgender issues but also sufficient competence to work in a respectful and appropriate way with a trans person in whatever program or capacity we might encounter them. We may find ourselves working with trans people as clients, co-workers or superiors in almost any setting and client population. We need to recognize any anxieties we may have regarding gender pronoun preference and, using our communications skills, inquire with clients at an appropriate time and in a respectful way; we are unlikely to be the first person to ask this of our clients who present as gender non-normative, but we might be the first to inquire respectfully.

As Hansbury (2005) cautions, many trans men are apprehensive about accessing service due to concerns about of mistreatment or inappropriate care, often based in their own lived experience. Therefore we need to consider how policies and procedures in our own practice or the programs we manage perpetuate the dominant "negative transition story." Further, we must be cautious that we are not making assumptions about trans clients' experiences being necessarily negative, problematic or even associated with being trans at all. As with gender pronouns, we have the opportunity to create new experiences for clients that are based in respect and dignity when we shape our interventions in terms of resilience and coping. As these stories have demonstrated, many trans clients have negotiated numerous systemic barriers and been forced to self-advocate for their healthcare.

There remains the need to consider the implication of being trans on more generic and mundane life experiences. For example, a trans man seeking medical attention for a broken arm may not require different medical treatment, but may still experience anxiety from the anticipation of being differently treated by health-care providers, even regardless of whether any mistreatment actually happens. The stress of anticipation or of needing to 'come out' as trans can make a mundane experience anxiety-provoking. By providing an environment where trans clients are welcomed respectfully and appropriately treated, we can help alleviate this anxiety. This environment can be created using strategies Pazos (1999) described earlier – increased cultural knowledge of trans communities, use of psycho-education, and understanding client resistance – and by recognizing that trans clients, like all clients, benefit from support, recognition and flexibility from service providers.

As the guys demonstrated, having resources, both financial and social, helped them maneuver through their transition process and the healthcare system more easily. When conducting strengths-based assessment, such as the pragmatic framework offered by Graybeal (2004), we can help our clients identify and nurture these resources. Beyond resources, we can investigate options clients have for their transition process that perhaps had heretofore gone unexplored. We can think creatively about what clients imagine for and of themselves once they meet their transition-related goals. In times when the realities of the "negative transition story" are manifest, we have the option to explore how they may continue to thrive through these challenges just as they have in the past. And we can invite clients to consider what they most want for themselves, and what they might dream about on Saturday mornings as they lay in bed.

At the same time there is a need to understand that gender transition happens in the context of other identities and marginalized categories such as race, age and sexual orientation. Further, due to a dominant sexuality discourse that problematically lumps trans people together with gay, lesbian and bisexual people, gender identity and sexual identity are commonly confused, resulting in an ever-present and on-going marginalization of trans people today. As providers we are well situated to help clients understand these issues, presenting us with a great opportunity to develop a deeper relationship.

Finally, providers who work with trans people in addictions can take insights from the stories shared here in order to understand that some degree of substance misuse may be directly related to trans clients' experiences of the "negative transition story." The tangible experiences of systemic barriers and social stigma can have an understandably detrimental impact on an individual's mental health and substances may be used in both helpful and unhelpful ways to cope with the resultant stress. With this understanding in mind, our role is to understand the societal contexts of our clients' struggles in relation to their personal life experiences.

Advanced clinical practice with trans men

For specialists in transgender healthcare there are a broader, more challenging and exciting array of practice issues that arise from this project. These men made their transition a priority and had the privilege to do so. Some paid out-of-pocket for surgery because they were not willing to give up power over their own medical transition process and to be put on a provincial-health-insurance waitlist. They recognized surgery was something they wanted and found a surgeon to do it. Keeping in mind what participants perceived as 'stuck in a middle place,' we can help clients assess any other concerns that might result in medical transition not being a primary interest for them. Not every trans person wants to, or is able to, prioritize transition as a foremost concern, so our assessment must also include awareness of clients' other priorities such as children and partners, competing health issues, and financial status.

Those people who are exploring their gender or considering transition may just listen at the door of the transition narrative and likely hear only the loudest voices sharing the "negative transition story." We have the opportunity to reframe that narrative and encourage clients to seek out other stories. To find positive stories took many months for some highly motivated participants, so we might refer clients to appropriate support groups where we know a balanced transition story is shared. Some might deny themselves transition and continue to live their lives while putting aside any thoughts of gender. The potential long-term negative impacts of denying gender identity on a person's mental health are a grave concern and may lead to depression, anxiety and unhelpful coping strategies like substance abuse. As mental health workers we should assess for these as possibilities and treat appropriately.

In terms of transition, we understand that some of our clients may just want HRT while others also want surgical interventions. There is no predestined end-point other than finding greater comfort with oneself. Our colleagues and other practitioners may struggle to understand clients for whom testosterone, surgeries and passing are not priorities. Gender transition is a personal journey, one that may, but does not need to, focus on the polar ends of the gender binary. Wherever our clients find themselves on the spectrum is fine, and wherever they are at today is just perfect even when there is a desire to change and grow.

Further, the men described the potential for making the transition experience an enjoyable one. The question being posed to trans and non-trans friends, allies and service providers is this: will we continue to perpetuate the "negative transition story" or will we instead encourage a journey that, while still fraught with real obstacles and challenges, can be pleasurable for the individual, leads to a more satisfied life, and makes a positive contribution to all communities?

It is my belief that the movement away from gender identity disorder as the central focus in trans health care is a litmus test for all providers: those who maintain that trans people are essentially mentally ill are not allies of trans people. As programs like Callen-Lorde Community Health Center in New York City demonstrate it is possible to move away from using GID/GD as the foundation of transition-related medical care in the United States (Douglass, 2009). Their *Informed Consent Model* puts the onus of responsibility and direction with the client and leaves the role of health providers to simply assess capacity for decision-making and provide ongoing advocacy and support.

Providers need to take a closer look at the assessment models currently used for trans people and move toward a more progressive and client-centred modality. We can explore options that might enable more clients to access the health care they desire. By shifting the focus away from treating transsexualism and toward helping our trans clients find a more comfortable way of being with themselves in their bodies, we end up with greater flexibility in our assessments and diagnoses. Any health-care intervention has the potential for generating stress related to disclosure and the potential for receiving treatment that is non-competent or explicitly transphobic. An additional challenge for service providers is to resist the assumption that GID/GD is the foundation of all health issues experienced by trans clients. Beyond the potential stress experienced by the client, it may be easier for us to recognize how treatment for a broken arm does not fall under the GID/GD umbrella of trans care; however it would be more challenging to assess chronic depression, anxiety, and dysthymic disorders that are clearly present in our trans clients, but not necessarily caused by or related to their being trans. The onus is on us as service providers to not take the easy diagnostic route. Can we imagine a clinical world where some of our clients may have mental illness and also, coincidentally, be trans?

As service providers, I believe we need to see the utility of using these findings to inform practice, and as a means of engaging with our clients in ways that we otherwise might not. It is possible that as a clinician I might never see people like those I interviewed. These trans men are not in need of our services and thus may never enter a clinic or program where a social worker is employed. By identifying an optimum state of well-being, and an end-goal for practice such as life satisfaction, I was able to learn about what that particular 'destination' might look like and, perhaps more importantly, understand better the journey. From here I can generate more informed, outcome-based goals with clients who may be starting and struggling with similar journeys.

In terms of working with trans men around addiction issues, some might think that concurrently broaching and even initiating transition would be foolhardy. As their stories underscored, engaging with trans men about their gender has the effect of reducing mental health symptoms. My recommendation would be that as practitioners the onus is on us to unpack and dismantle the "negative transition story" during counseling in order to de-escalate any possible triggers or concerns our clients may have. In the next chapter I offer the framework for doing so.

6 | AN ASSESSMENT TOOL FOR
TRANSGENDER-RELATED STRESS & TRAUMA

Mental health concerns like depression, anxiety and substance abuse experienced by a trans person may or may not be related to gender identity issues, particularly when those concerns involve societal oppression. As previously stated by Lev (2004), one of the reasons trans clients seek help is to address gender-related distress. She argues that the fear trans people have for transgressing normative gender behaviours, and the long-term performance of a false self may actually cause mental health issues (p.196):

> The high incidence of mental illness among transgendered people noted in the literature might be better understood as reactive symptomology and posttraumatic sequalae. It is literally *crazy-making* to live a false self. (p.196, original emphasis)

Lev suggests that these illnesses might actually be expressions of deep-seated trauma. This approach reveals transgenderism and 'Gender Identity Disorder' as expressions of mental health symptoms and substitutes these with an etiological view of Post-Traumatic Stress Disorder (PTSD). PTSD is another *DSM* diagnosis familiar to practitioners that comes without the burden of the gender-related stigma. The key then, if the foundations of transgender mental health are based in PTSD, is for service providers to explore these issues with their trans clients in order to provide effective treatment.

This Assessment Tool is intended for use by social workers, counselors, and other healthcare clinicians who assess or treat transgender men and other gender non-conforming people with regard to mental health and wellness. Wherever clients are in their transition journeys, this tool is intended help professionals create an environment where trans individuals can explore their experiences. Peer counselors and group facilitators may also find it useful.

Why is this tool important?

Many trans people are not open about their gender identity in mainstream treatment and counseling facilities for fear of maltreatment or negative attitudes from staff and other clients (Raj, 2002). Programs for trans men and gender-variant people need evidence-based tools to help assess and support individuals during and after transition. Even clinicians with a strong understanding of gender identity issues may lack a repertoire of appropriate questions to ask about gender identity. Others may be unaware of why such questions are necessary for clients of substance abuse and/or mental health services.

Emergent life factors

Trans men I spoke with identified specific life factors that related to their mental health and wellness. Transition-related concerns included: medical (hormones and surgeries) and non-medical transition options; 'passing' and being read as their affirmed gender; trans-related 'coming out' to partners, friends and family, and concerns about loss of support; societal oppression due to transphobia; threats to socioeconomic security (e.g., housing, employment) because of discrimination; isolation and alienation; and internalized oppression. Non-transition-related issues identified by participants included: body image; concerns with aging; substance abuse and recovery; dating and relationships with non-trans people (heterosexual, lesbian and queer women, gay and queer men); sexual intimacy issues; and concerns about long-term use of hormones.

Awareness of unresolved issues stemming from transition is vital to effective treatment and counseling. Until now the impacts of transition-related stress and trauma have not been adequately described (Lev, 2004), nor have interventions been created to effectively address these. By using this tool, counselors have the opportunity to develop deeper rapport by identifying and supporting issues that are unique to the transition experience. While this tool was developed based on evidence from a research project focused on trans men, counselors working with trans women may also find this helpful.

Assessment tool questions

This assessment tool includes a set of six open-ended interview items to be asked by the counselor during assessment or group process. These questions are informed by a strengths-based model commonly used in social work practice (for a primer on strengths-based practice, see Graybeal, 2004). Questions were crafted using culturally-specific and trans-affirming language for engagement with trans people, and designed to be asked in a particular order. While counselors and facilitators will use their own style, the rationale for each question explains the important elements of each.

AN ASSESSMENT TOOL FOR TRANSGENDER-RELATED STRESS AND TRAUMA

© Marcus Greatheart MSW

1. Identify transition-related narratives

- What are the stories you have heard about transition?
- How accurate are/were those stories?
- How much influence do/did you have in shifting those stories?
- How do/did you experience your power?

2. Contextualize hormones and surgeries among other transition-related options

- What do/did you see as the options for transition?
- What options do/did you want, what are/were you considering, and what do/did you not want for yourself?
- What significance do/did or don't/didn't hormones and surgeries have in your transition experience?
- Setting aside hormones and surgeries, what are/were the important milestones on your journey?

3. Identify key social supports and their contributions

- Which supports are/were most helpful in your transition?
- In what way were they helpful?

4. Illustrate capacity for self-efficacy

- What strategies do/did you use to manage any barriers or challenges you experienced?

5. Unpack the emotional impacts of privilege or disadvantage

- What opportunities have/did you take/n advantage of to further your transition?
- What feelings do you attach to these?

6. Create tangible strategies to generate new transition narratives

- What is it about your transition story that might be helpful for other trans men to hear?
- How might you go about sharing your transition story in a concrete way that benefits other trans men?

QUESTION 1: Identify transition-related narratives

These questions begin the process of storytelling and help individuals unpack the competing and likely difficult components of the transition narrative including the "negative transition story" described in this book. Clients assess these stories and situate themselves within these narratives as subjective entities.

QUESTION 2: Contextualize hormones and surgeries among other transition-related options

Clients begin to explore the menu of options that transition has available. Many will see HRT and surgeries as the foundations for their transition experience. The intention is to look at what components individuals include in their visions of gender transition, including changes to the body that may make living in it more comfortable. Medically-mediated gender reassignment interventions are contextualized over a broader realm of choices. The importance of being 'read' as the affirmed gender and the understanding of potential biological and genetic limitations to doing so are explored.

By asking what clients do and do not want creates an opportunity to explore their decision-making process and feelings related to each option. The final question asks clients to set aside hormones and surgery specifically, thereby revealing how the dominant transition narrative tends to foreground these interventions. This gives the practitioner the opportunity to investigate with clients what other significant events and experiences impacted their transition. In this way we begin to poke holes in the dominant narrative and allow a new and personalized transition story to emerge.

QUESTION 3: Identify key social supports and their contributions

With these questions individuals can speak about the social supports that are important to them, and qualify how these relationships are made meaningful. They discuss the specific actions and events, and the insights they may have in relation to these.

QUESTION 4: Illustrate capacity for self-efficacy

With these questions, clients explore specific instances where they demonstrated resilience, and how these previous experiences confirmed the client's ability to cope with the challenges they may face in the future.

QUESTION 5: Unpacking the emotional impacts of privilege or disadvantage

By discussing how they mobilized any privilege they experienced, clients demonstrate self-efficacy but may also reveal unexpressed emotions like guilt or anger toward their social networks, trans and broader communities. This question may be the climax of the narrative and therefore open the deepest emotions.

Question 6 - Creating tangible strategies to generate new transition narratives.

Finally, clients have the opportunity to consider, in the context of problematic narratives, that they can create new ones. Further, they can act on these in tangible ways.

I invite your feedback on this *Assessment Tool*. My hope is that this framework will grow organically as practitioners use it.
I will incorporate feedback and make revisions available through the book's website at www.TransformingPractice.net.

7 | FINAL THOUGHTS

Transition is not the journey: life satisfaction is. On the road to satisfaction there is a stretch of highway that involves coming to terms with one's body. I hope that this book has provided some valuable insights into the description of a problematic dominant narrative about transition and the highly problematic impacts of this discourse on the everyday lives of these participants. Trans men can have both enjoyable transition experiences and lead contented lives. I am convinced that my role as an ally and health provider is to break down the "negative transition story" and remind my trans men friends and clients of a better, more positive and fulfilling opportunity to transition in a way that foregrounds the personal and social over the medical, and leads to an overall more enjoyable experience for the individual, his family, friends and supporters.

8 | REFERENCES

American Psychiatric Association. (2000). *Diagnostic and statistical manual of mental disorders: DSM-IV-TR* (4th , text revision ed.). Washington, DC: American Psychiatric Association.

American Psychological Association. *Answers to your questions about transgender individuals and gender identity.* Retrieved 15 November 2012 from http://www.apa.org/topics/transgender.html.

Barbara, A. M., Chaim, G., Doctor, F., & Centre for Addiction and Mental Health. (2007). *Asking the right questions, 2: Talking with clients about sexual orientation and gender identity in mental health, counselling and addiction settings* (Rev. ed.). Toronto: Centre for Addiction and Mental Health.

Benjamin, H. (1966). *The transsexual phenomenon.* New York, N.Y: Julian Press.

Bockting, W., Knudson, G. & Goldberg, J. (2006). *Endocrine therapy for transgender adults in British Columbia: Suggested guidelines - assessment of hormone eligibility and readiness*. Retrieved 115 November 2012 from http://transhealth.vch.ca/resources/.

Bockting, W. O., Robinson, B. E., & Rosser, B. R. S. (1998). Transgender HIV prevention: A qualitative needs assessment. *AIDS Care, 10*(4), 505-525.

Brill, S. (2009, 04 September) Provider's seminar: Working with transgender and gender-variant children and youth. Presented at the Gender Odyssey Conference, Seattle, WA.

British Columbia Association of Social Workers (BCASW). (2003). *Code of ethics*. Retrieved 15 November 2012 from http://www.bcasw.org/about-bcasw/casw-code-of-ethics/

Canadian Mental Health Association. Retrieved 15 November 2012 from http://www.cmha.ca

Carroll, L., & Gilroy, P. J. (2002). Transgender issues in counselor preparation. *Counselor Education & Supervision, 41*(3), 233.

CBC News. (2009). *Transgendered Albertans file human-rights complaints*. Retrieved 15 November 2012 from http://www.cbc.ca/canada/calgary/story/2009/04/15/cgy-alberta-transgendered-sex-change-human-rights.html.

Chekola, M. (1974). *The concept of happiness*. Unpublished Doctoral thesis, University of Michigan.

Clements-Nolle, K., Marx, R., & Katz, M. (2006). Attempted suicide among transgender persons: The influence of gender-based discrimination and victimization. *Journal of Homosexuality,* *51*(3), 53-69.

Cohen-Kettenis, P., & Pfäfflin, F. (2009). *The DSM diagnostic criteria for gender identity disorder in adolescents and adults.* *Archives of Sexual Behavior (39(2),* 499-513.

Cole, S., Denny, D., Eyler, A. E., & Samons, S. (2000). Issues of transgender. In L. T. Szuchman, & F. Muscarella (Eds.), *Psychological perspectives on human sexuality* (pp. 149-195). New York, NY: Wiley.

Cole, C. M., O'Boyle, M., Emory, L. E., & Meyer III, W. J. (1997). Comorbidity of gender dysphoria and other major psychiatric diagnoses. *Archives of Sexual Behavior, 26*(1), 13-26.

Conway, L. (2002). *Estimating the prevalence of transsexualism.* Retrieved 20 November 2012 from http://ai.eecs.umich.edu/people/conway/TS/TSprevalence.html.

Cousins, N. (1989). *Head first: The biology of hope* (1st ed.). New York, NY: Dutton.

CPATH (2011, Fall). Provincial Updates. *Canadian Professional Association for Trangender Health Newsletter, Vol. 23.* Retrieved from http://www.cpath-fall-2011-newsletter-Nov-22-14H35.pdf

Cuypere, G., Jannes, C., & Rubens, R. (1995). Psychosocial functioning of transsexuals in Belgium. *Acta Psychiatrica Scandinavica, 91*(3), 180-184.

Devor, A. H. (2004). Witnessing and mirroring: A fourteen stage model of transsexual identity formation. *Journal of Gay & Lesbian Psychotherapy, 8*(1), 41-67.

Devor, A.H. (1997) FTM: Female-to-male transsexuals in society. Bloomington, IN: Indiana University Press.

dickey, l. m. (2009, 05 September). Female-to-male transsexuals: A literature review. Presented at the Gender Odyssey Conference, Seattle, WA.

Diener, E. (1984). Subjective well-being. *Psychological Bulletin, 95*(3), 542-575.

Douglass, K. (2009, 10 June). Alternatives to gender identity as a diagnosis for health and mental health care providers. Presented at the Philadelphia Trans Health Conference, Philadelphia, PA.

Drescher, J. (2009). Queer diagnoses: Parallels and contrasts in the history of homosexuality, gender variance, and the diagnostic and statistical manual. *Archives of Sexual Behavior, 39*(2), 427-460.

Edelman, E. A. (2009). The power of stealth: (in)visible site of female-to-male transsexual resistance. In E. Lewin, & W. Leap (Eds.), *Out in public: Reinventing Lesbian/Gay anthropology in a globalizing world* (pp. 164-179-365). Chichester, U.K.: Wiley-Blackwell.

Ekins, R., & King, D. (1999). Towards sociology of transgendered bodies. *Sociological Review, 47*(3), 580-602.

Forshee, A. (2008). Transgender men: A demographic snapshot. *Journal of Gay & Lesbian Social Services, 20*(3), 221-236.

Goldberg, J., Matte, N., MacMillan, M., & Hudspith, M. J. (2003). *VCHA/Community survey: Transition/crossdressing services in BC - final.* Vancouver: Vancouver Coastal Health Authority. Retrieved 29 November, 2012 from http://transhealth.vch.ca/.

Graybeal, C. (2004). Strengths-based social work assessment: Transforming the dominant paradigm. *Families in Society, 82*(3), 233-242.

Green, J. (2009, 25 September). TransMen's sexual practices and sexual health. Presented at the Southern Comfort Conference, Atlanta, GA.

Hansbury, G. (2005). The middle men. *Studies in Gender & Sexuality, 6*(3), 241-264.

Harding, K. M. D., & Feldman, M. M. D. (2006). Transgender emergence: Therapeutic guidelines for working with gender-variant people and their families. *Journal of the American Academy of Child & Adolescent Psychiatry, 45*(5), 627-630.

Healy, K. (2001). Participatory action research and social work: A critical appraisal. *International Social Work, 44*(1), 93-105.

Hembree, W. C., Cohen-Kettenis, P., Delemarre-van de Waal, H. A., Gooren, L. J., Meyer, W. J.,III, Spack, N. P., et al. (2009). Endocrine treatment of transsexual persons: An endocrine society clinical practice guideline. *Journal of Clinical Endocrinology Metabolism, 94*(9), 3132-3154.

Hird, M. J. (2000). Gender's nature: Intersexuality, transsexualism and the 'sex'/'gender' binary. *Feminist Theory, 1*(3), 347-364.

Holman, C. W., & Goldberg, J. M. (2006). Social and medical transgender case advocacy. *International Journal of Transgenderism, 9*(3), 197-217.

Hughes, T. L., & Eliason, M. (2002). Substance use and abuse in lesbian, gay, bisexual and transgender populations. *The Journal of Primary Prevention, 22*(3), 263-298.

International Lesbian, Gay, Bisexual, Trans and Intersex Association Trans Secretariat. (2009). *Transsexualism will no longer be classified as a mental illness in France.* Retrieved 10/25/2012 from http://trans.ilga.org/trans/welcome_to_the_ilga_trans_secretaria t/news/france_transsexualism_will_no_longer_be_classified_as_ a_mental_illness_in_france.

Joseph, S., & Linley, P. A. (2005). Positive adjustment to threatening events: An organismic valuing theory of growth through adversity. *Review of General Psychology, 9*(3), 262-280.

Kenagy, G. P. (2002). HIV among transgendered people. *AIDS Care, 14*(1), 127-134.

Kenagy, G. P., & Hsieh, C. (2005). The risk less known: Female-to-male transgender persons' vulnerability to HIV infection. *AIDS Care, 17*(2), 195-207.

Knudson, G., & Corneil, T. (2009, November 12). *Access to surgical care across Canada (personal communication)*.

Krueger, R. A., & Casey, M. A. (2009). *Focus groups: A practical guide for applied research* (4th ed.). Los Angeles, CA: SAGE.

Lawrence, A. (2007). Transgender health concerns. In I. H. Meyer, & M. E. Northridge (Eds.), *The health of sexual minorities: Public health perspectives on lesbian, gay, bisexual and transgender populations* (pp. 473-505). New York, NY: Springer.

Lev, A. I. (2004). *Transgender emergence: Therapeutic guidelines for working with gender-variant people and their families.* New York, NY: The Haworth Clinical Practice Press.

Lobato, M. I., Koff, W. J., Manenti, C., da, F. S., Salvador, J., et al. (2006). Follow-up of sex reassignment surgery in transsexuals: A Brazilian cohort. *Archives of Sexual Behavior, 35*(6), 711-715.

Lorber, J. (2005). *Gender inequality: Feminist theories and politics* (3rd ed.). Los Angeles, CA: Roxbury Pub.

Maguen, S., Shipherd, J. C., & Harris, H. N. (2005). Providing culturally sensitive care for transgender patients. *Cognitive and Behavioral Practice, 12*(4), 479-490.

Maton, K. I. (2004). *Investing in children, youth, families, and communities: Strengths-based research and policy.* Washington, DC: APA Books.

Meier, S. C., & Fitzgerald, K. (2009, 06 September). The positive effects of hormonal gender affirmation treatment on mental health in female to male transsexuals. Presented at the Gender Odyssey Conference, Seattle, WA.

Meyer, W., Bockting, W. O., Cohen-Kettenis, P., Coleman, E., DiCeglie, D., Devor, H., Gooren, L., Hage, J., Kirk, S., Kuiper, B., Laub, D., Lawrence, A., Menard, Y., Patton, J., Schaefer, L., Webb, A. & Wheeler, C.C. (2001). The Harry Benjamin International Gender Dysphoria Association's *Standards of Care for Gender Identity Disorders*, sixth version. *Journal of Psychology & Human Sexuality, 13*(1), 1.

Monro, S., & Warren, L. (2004). Transgendering citizenship. *Sexualities, 7*(3), 345-362.

National Association of Social Workers. (2008). *Code of ethics.* Retrieved October 27, 2012 from http://www.socialworkers.org.

Newfield, E., Hart, S., Dibble, S., & Kohler, L. (2006). Female-to-male transgender quality of life. *Quality of Life Research: An International Journal of Quality of Life Aspects of Treatment, Care and Rehabilitation, 15*(9), 1447-1457.

O'Neill, B. (2002). '...We didn't connect at all...': The experiences of a gay client. *Journal of Gay & Lesbian Social Services. 14*(4), 75-91.

Pazos, S. (1999). Practice with female-to-male transgender youth. *Journal of Gay & Lesbian Social Services, 10*(3/4), 65-82.

Pennebaker, J. W., & Seagal, J. D. (1999). Forming a story: The health benefits of narrative. *Journal of Clinical Psychology, 55*(10), 1243-1254.

Potts, K., & Brown, L. (2005). *Research as resistance: Critical, indigenous and anti-oppressive approaches.* Toronto, ON: Canadian Scholars' Press.

Radley, A. (1990). Artifacts, memory and a sense of the past. In D. Middleton, & D. Edwards (Eds.), *Collective remembering* (pp. 46-59). Newbury Park, CA: Sage Publications.

Raj, R. (2002). Towards a transpositive therapeutic model: Developing clinical sensitivity and cultural competence in the effective support of transsexual and transgendered clients. *International Journal of Transgenderism, 6*(2).

Raymond, J. G. (1979). *The transsexual empire: The making of the she-male.* Boston, MA: Beacon Press.

Raymond, J. G. (1994). The politics of transgender. *Feminism & Psychology, 4*(4), 628-633.

Riaño Alcalá, P. (2004). Encounters with memory and mourning: Public art as collective pedagogy of reconciliation. In J. F. Ibáñez-Carrasco, & E. R. Meiners (Eds.), *Public acts: Disruptive readings on making curriculum public* (pp. 211-230). New York, NY: RoutledgeFalmer.

Riaño Alcalá, P. (2006). *Dwellers of memory: Youth and violence in Medellín, Colombia.* New Brunswick, N.J: Transaction Publishers.

Rothberg, P. *The DSM-V and Kenneth Zucker.* Retrieved October 25, 2012, from http://www.thenation.com/blog/dsm-v-and-kenneth-zucker

Ryff, C. D. (1989). Happiness is everything, or is it? Explorations on the meaning of psychological well-being. *Journal of Personality and Social Psychology, 57*(6), 1069-1081.

Salamon, G. (2005). Transmasculinity and relation commentary on Griffin Hansbury's "middle men." *Studies in Gender & Sexuality, 6*(3), 265-275.

Saleebey, D. (1996). The strengths perspective in social work practice: Extensions and cautions. *Social Work, 41*(3), 296-305.

Scanlon, K. (2006). Where's the beef: Masculinity as performed by feminists. In K. Scott-Dixon (Ed.), *Trans/Forming feminisms: Trans-feminist voices speak out* (pp. 87-94). Toronto, ON: Sumach Press.

Scott, R. (Director). (1991). *Thelma & Louise.* [Motion Picture].

Scott-Dixon, K. (Ed.). (2006). *Trans/Forming feminisms: Trans-feminist voices speak out.* Toronto, ON: Sumach Press.

Seil, D. (2004). The diagnosis and treatment of transgendered patients. *Journal of Gay & Lesbian Psychotherapy, 8*(1), 99.

Serano, J. (2009, June 17). Keynote: Psychology, sexualization, and trans-invalidations. *Philadelphia Trans Health Conference,* Philadelphia, PA.

Shin, D. C., & Johnson, D. M. (1978). Avowed happiness as an overall assessment of the quality of life. *Social Indicators Research, 5*(4), 475.

Smit, E. (2006). Western psychiatry and gender identity disorder (GID): A critical perspective. In F. Boonzaaier, & P. Kiguwa (Eds.), *The gender of psychology* (pp. 250-292). Cape Town, South Africa: Juta.

Stryker, S. (2008). *Transgender history.* Berkeley, CA: Seal Press

Substance Abuse and Mental Health Services Administration. (2001). *A Provider's introduction to substance abuse treatment for lesbian, gay, bisexual, and transgender individuals.* Rockville,

MD: US Department of Health and Human Services. Retrieved 15 Nov 2012 from http://www.kap.samhsa.gov/products/manuals/pdfs/lgbt.pdf.

Taylor, E. (2006). *Untitled.* Unpublished MSW graduating essay, School of Social Work, University of British Columbia.

La transsexualité ne sera plus classée maladie mentale. (2009, May 18) *Le Figaro,* pp. n.p. Retrieved September 29, 2012 from http://www.lefigaro.fr/sante/2009/05/18/01004-20090518ARTFIG00386-la-transsexualite-ne-sera-plus-classee-maladie-mentale-.php.

van Kesteren, P. J. M., Asscheman, H., Megens, J. A. J., & Gooren, L. J. G. (1997). Mortality and morbidity in transsexual subjects treated with cross-sex hormones. *Clinical Endocrinology, 47*(3), 337-343.

Vancouver Coastal Health. *Transgender health program.* Retrieved November 30, 2012 from http://transhealth.vch.ca/.

Verschoor, A. M., & Poortinga, J. (1988). Psychosocial differences between Dutch male and female transsexuals. *Archives of Sexual Behavior, 17*(2), 173-178.

Vital Statistics Act, 27 (1996). British Columbia, Canada. Retrieved December 02, 2012 from http://www.bclaws.ca/EPLibraries/bclaws_new/document/ID/freeside/00_96479_01#section27

Wilson, A. (2005, November 9). Transgender health benefits: Getting coverage through policy change. Paper presented at *National Gay and Lesbian Task Force Creating Change Conference*. Oakland, CA.

World Health Organization. (1990). *International classification of diseases (ICD, 2nd edition*. Retrieved 15 November 2012 from http://www.who.int/classifications/icd/en/index.html.

WPATH standards of care. (2011). Retrieved 15 November 2012 from http://www.wpath.org/publications_standards.cfm.

ABOUT THE AUTHOR

Marcus Greatheart is a trans ally, author, speaker and social worker in private practice. He provides counselling, workshops and conference presentations with a focus on sexuality and gender. This includes individuals and couples on the lesbian, gay and bisexual spectrum; trans people and those questioning their gender; kinky people, and those who are in alternative and polyamorous relationships.

Marcus has more than 20 years' experience in community health, particularly sexual health and HIV. He has a BA (History in Art) from the University of Victoria, BC, and a Master of Social Work from the University of British Columbia. He currently attends the Michael de Groote School of Medicine at McMaster University and lives in the Niagara Region of Ontario. Find him online at www.greatheart.ca.

TransformingPractice.net

- Bonus Material
- Curated resource lists for providers, researchers & community members
- Feedback on the *Assessment Tool for Transgender-related Stress and Trauma*
- Latest Blog entries by the author

Send us your transition stories!

We heard loud and clear that positive, affirming, and hope-filled stories of gender transition are helpful to those struggling or just getting started.

So we're building an online community space where post-transition trans people can share experiences that might help others along their journey.

Health Providers can invite their clients to submit their stories. It benefits the community on the whole, and we believe sharing our stories offers positive therapeutic benefit.

Send us short stories that describe a pivotal moment in transition, along with photos, artwork and other images that complement the narrative.

TransitionStories.org